# Fundamentals of Health and Physical Education

**Joe Eshuys**
**Vic Guest**
**Judith Lawrence**
Coleen Jackson
Dee Bunnage

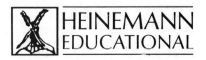
HEINEMANN
EDUCATIONAL

Heinemann Educational
a division of Heinemann Educational Books Ltd,
Halley Court, Jordan Hill, Oxford 0X2 8EJ

OXFORD  LONDON  EDINBURGH
MADRID  ATHENS  BOLOGNA  PARIS
MELBOURNE  SYDNEY  AUCKLAND  SINGAPORE  TOKYO
IBADAN  NIAROBI  HARARE  GABORONE
PORTSMOUTH NH (USA)

First published in 1987 by The Jacaranda Press
33 Park Road, Milton, Queensland, Australia 4064
New material © Heinemann Educational 1990

**British Library Cataloguing in Publication Data**
Fundamentals of Health and Physical Education –
Rev. ed.
  1. Physical Education
  I Eshuys, Joe

613.7

ISBN 0 435 13000 5

Illustrated by Mandy Cilento

Cover photograph by Robert Harding Picture Library

Printed in Great Britain
by Scotprint Ltd, Musselburgh

91 92 93 94 95    12 11 10 9 8 7 6 5 4 3

**Some exercises can cause injury, especially
if they are attempted before achieving an
appropriate level of physical fitness. We
therefore advise the reader to seek medical
advice before beginning a programme of
exercises or attempting any of the exercises
described in this book. Neither the
publisher nor the authors can accept
responsibility for any injury that might be
sustained when performing any of the
exercises or procedures described in this
book.**

# Contents

**Acknowledgements** vi

**Unit A  Studying Health and Physical Education  1**

    **1. What is Health and Physical Education?  2**

      The history of Health and Physical Education 2
      Health and Physical Education today 3

**Unit B  Foundations of physical education  11**

    **2. Your body  12**

      The human body 12
        What is the body made of? 12/ Systems of
        the body 12
      The skeletal system 14
        The functions of the skeletal system 14/
        The structure and workings of the skeletal
        system 14/ joints 16/ connective tissue 19
      The muscular system 19
        The functions of the muscular system 19/
        The structure and workings of the muscular
        system 19
      The circulatory system 23
        The functions of the circulatory system 24/
        The structure and workings of the
        circulatory system 24
      The respiratory system 28
        The functions of the respiratory system 28/
        The structure and workings of the
        respiratory system 29/ Breathing 30
      The digestive system 31
        The functions of the digestive system 31/
        The structure and workings of the digestive
        system 32
      The excretory system 34
        The functions of the excretory system 34/
        The structure and workings of the excretory
        system 34

The nervous system 35
    The functions of the nervous system 35/
    The structure and workings of the nervous
    system 35
The endocrine system 38
    The functions of the endocrine system 38/
    The structure and workings of the endocrine
    system 39
The skin system 40
    The functions of the skin system 40/
    The structure and workings of the skin
    system 41

## 3. The body in movement  42

Movement 42
    Systems working together 42/ The action of
    muscles 42/ Joints 42/ Naming movement 43/
    Factors affecting movement 47/ Motion 54
The use of momentum and motion 58
    Stopping an object 59
Posture 59
    Good posture when standing 59/ Good
    posture when sitting 60/ Good posture when
    walking 61/ Importance of the feet 61/
    Lifting posture 62

## 4. Fitness and performance  63

The components of fitness 63
    Endurance 64/ Strength 65/ Flexibility 65/
    Power 65/ Speed 66/ Agility, balance,
    reaction time and coordination 66
Assessing and improving your fitness level 68
    Cardio-vascular endurance 68/ Muscular
    endurance 72/ Strength 74/ Flexibility 77/
    Power 84/ Speed 85/ Agility, balance,
    reaction time and coordination 85
Training for performance 88
    The warm-up 88/ The training activities 89/
    The cool-down 91
Food for fitness 92
    Water 92/ Protein 92/ Carbohydrates 92/
    Fats 93/ Vitamins and minerals 93/ Eating
    and competing 93

## 5. Sports injuries and their prevention  95

The causes of sports injuries 96
    External causes 96/ Internal causes 97
Prevention of sports injuries 97
    Knowledge of your body 97/ Player
    suitability 99/ Training methods 99/
    Protective equipment 100/ The rules of the
    game 101/ Facilities 102/
Injuries in sport 102
    Procedure in the case of an injury 102

Common sports injuries 104
  Soft tissue injuries 104/ Hard tissue
  injuries 108/ Joint injuries 109/ Other
  common injuries 111
Rehabilitation 113

### 6. Sport, society and you  114
Development of sport 114
The sociology of sport 115
  What is sport? 115
People and sport 118
  The players 118/ The officials 121/
  Spectators 122/ sponsors 125/
Other issues in sport 127
  Professionalism 127/ Sport and politics 127/
  Sport and terrorism 128/ Sport and
  women 128/ Sport and disabled people 130/
  Drugs and sport 131
Changing views 132

## Unit C  Health

### 7. Health and you  136
What is health? 136
Physical well-being 136
  What is physical fitness? 136/ Why be fit? 136/
  Becoming physically fit 137

### 8. Health and diet  138
What are nutrients? 138
Nutrients in your diet 138
  Carbohydrates 138/ Proteins 139/ Fats and
  oils 139/ Vitamins 139/ Minerals 141/ Water
  and fibre 141
A balanced diet 143
  The six food groups 144/ Weight
  control 145

### 9. Drugs and your health  147
What are drugs? 147
  Smoking 147/ Drinking 149
Drugs 150
Anabolic steroids 151
Pressures of sport 152

### Index  153

# Acknowledgements

The authors would like to give particular thanks to their consultants, Howard Toyne, Cliff Mallett and Liz Sinclair.

They would also like to recognise the advice of Dr Andrew Graham and Dr Richard Pearson on the anatomy and biomechanics chapters, and acknowledge Stirling Buchanan, D.C., for his review of the chapter on sports injuries. The authors also acknowledge the advice of Richard Johnson, and the assistance given by the following physical educators: Rhonda Gray, Linda Guiness, Sue and Steve Harrold, Sue Kassulke, Rod Lennox, Graeme McGill, Peter Marconi, Bill Martin, Danny Mauro, John Nunan, Rita O'Neil and Jim Williams.

## Photo credits:

Ronald Sheridan's Photo Library, p. 3; Australian Associated Press, pp. 8 (bottom), 44, 57, 91, 92, 118 (left); Queensland Newspapers, pp. 11, 48, 50, 55, 64 (left), 65, 67, 85, 98, 100 (right), 101 (left), 105, 108, 112, 116 (left), 117 (top), 119 (right), 120, 122, 124 (bottom left), 126, 127, 130, 132, 146, UPI/Bettmann Newsphotos, pp. 9 (bottom right), 10 (left); Associated Press, pp. 49, 53, 66 (bottom right), 108, 109, 111 (bottom), 119 (left), 124 (bottom right), 128; INP-Photo, pp. 54, 118 (right); West Australian Newspapers, p. 88; Herald and Weekly Times, pp. 113, 121; London Express, p. 124 (top); Peter Bull, pp. 66 (top right), 129 (right); Sue Colquhoun, p. 72; Peter Ward, pp. 99 (left), 129 (bottom left); Gary Moore, pp. 1, 79; Peter McGrath, p. 19; Geoff Potter Photography, pp. 75, 77, 83; G. Guest, pp. 111 (top), 115, 131, Glen Watson, p. 117 (bottom); Allaction, pp. 66, 95, 99, 101; Allsport, pp. 50, 64, 95; Allsport/Duffy, pp. 9, 97; Barnabys Picture Library, p. 71; Colorsport, pp. 1, 71, 100; Chris Ridgers, p. 143.

## Other:

Table 1.1 BBC Sports Library; Figure 2.1 after G. Tortora and N. P. Anagnostakos, *Principles of Anatomy and Physiology*, 2nd ed. (San Francisco: Canfield Press, 1978); figure 2.3 after Jacob, Francone and Lossow, *Structure and Function in Man*, 4th ed. (Philadelphia: Saunders, 1978); figures 2.4 and 2.29 after William F. Evans, *Anatomy and Physiology*, 2nd ed. (Englewood Cliffs: Prentice Hall, 1971); figures 2.21-2.24 after David Allbrook, *How Bodies Work* (Brisbane: Jacaranda, 1979); figure 2.38 after Barnard, *The Body Machine* (London: Hamlyn, 1981); figure 2.40 after Bishop et al., *Science for Life* (London: Collins, 1984); figures 3.28-3.32 *Creating Posture Awareness*, Division of Health Education and Information; figure 4.2 after Charles Corbin and Ruth Lindsay, *Fitness for Life*, 2nd ed. (Glenview: Scott, Foresman, 1983); data for graphs in figures 4.1, 4.3, 4.6, 4.12 and 8.2 from *Australian Health and Fitness Survey 1985*, Australian Council for Health, Physical Education and Recreation, Inc.; p. 133 after Telecom Australia; figure 8.1 after Australian Nutrition Foundation; figure 9.2 after E. Goddard: Smoking Among Secondary School Children in England, 1988, HMSO, 1989; The Health Education Authority as the registered holder of the logo on page 134; The Sports Council as the registered holder of the logos on page 135.

# Unit A

## Studying Health and Physical Education

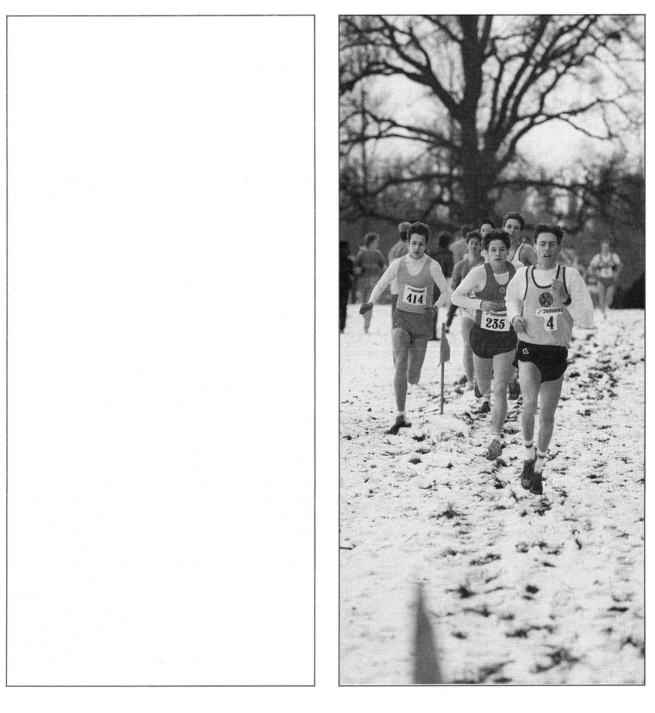

# 1

# What is Health and Physical Education?

Health and Physical Education is a study to provide you with information and practical experiences that will help you to make decisions about your physical, mental and social well-being.

## The history of Health and Physical Education

Health and Physical Education, in one form or another, has been an important part of people's lives throughout the ages.

- During the Stone Ages, people had to be fit to survive. An important physical activity was dance, which was practised at religious ceremonies, and used for entertainment and teaching.
- In ancient Sumer and Egypt, wrestling and other sports were encouraged, and dancing was very popular at festivals and religious ceremonies.
- In ancient China, exercise and meditation were practised for fitness and health.
- In ancient Greece, especially in Athens, education stressed the development of the whole person, both the body and the mind. Thus, besides citizenship, public speaking, history, mathematics, science, poetry and music, Greek boys learned physical activities such as jumping, running, boxing, wrestling, and throwing the javelin and discus. As well as keeping them fit and healthy, the Greeks saw these sports as

useful for basic military training. Dance continued to be an important part of Greek life. However, we remember the Greeks most as the people who began the Olympic Games. Originally, the Games were set up as a religious festival to honour the gods of Mount Olympus. The Games introduced three important developments:
  - *Spectators*. Huge crowds of spectators attended the Games. At the ancient Olympics, however, only men were allowed to watch and compete.
  - *Full-time athletes*. Competition became more intense forcing athletes to try for higher and higher standards. This meant that athletes had to spend much of their time training; the idea of the full-time athlete began to develop.
  - *Sporting hero*. Successful athletes won great glory. The idea of the "sporting hero" was born.
- In ancient Rome, sport was a part of a boy's education. Again, sports which would help in later army life were the most popular — ball games, throwing games, boxing, running, wrestling, swimming and horse-riding. Like the Greeks, many Romans kept healthy by eating a balanced diet and by being hygienic.

The ancient Romans further developed spectator sports for entertainment. Huge stadiums were built to hold great crowds who came to watch chariot racing and the cruel and bloody gladiatorial shows. The best gladiators and chariot drivers became "sporting heroes".

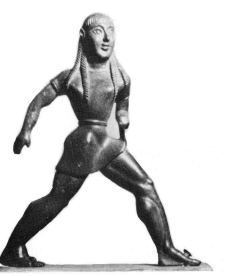

A bronze statuette of a runner in the starting position, c. 480–470 B.C.

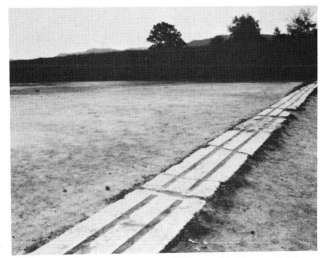

The starting line in the stadium at Olympia, where the ancient Games were held.

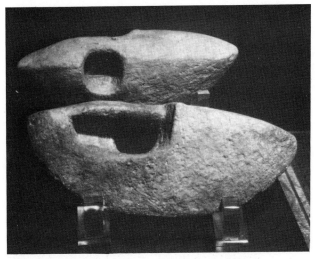

An athlete's hand-held jumping weight.

- During the Middle Ages, the sons of noble families were trained in physical activities to develop the skills of war. They learned swimming, wrestling, horseriding, hunting and fighting skills.
- During the Renaissance, people returned to the ideas of ancient Greece and Rome and once more stressed the need for education in mind and body. Ancient sports were taught and ball games with bats or racquets also became popular.
- Through the seventeenth, eighteenth and nineteenth centuries, physical education continued to be important. Often, physical education in schools was seen as a way to reinforce moral and religious ideas, to develop team spirit and to encourage the development of good character. New activities such as gymnastics and orienteering were introduced.
- By the twentieth century, Health and Physical Education continued to be an important part of school life. However, as knowledge in science and medicine grew, educators realised that students needed to increase their understanding of the theory of Health and Physical Education.

# Health and Physical Education today

The study of Health and Physical Education continues to be important because people want to:
- be healthy
- learn about their bodies
- learn about different sports
- learn about a wide range of recreational activities.

One method of studying Health and Physical Education is to divide it into three areas:
- *Foundations of physical education.* This covers how the body works and moves and methods to improve levels of performance. It also includes the roles and attitudes of people in games and sports.

- *Health.* This helps you to make decisions about maintaining and improving your health.
- *Games and sports.* This provides the knowledge and skills required in a wide range of physical activities.

In this book we are concerned with the first two areas: Foundations of Physical Education and Health.

# The modern Olympic Games

## History

The origin of the ancient Greek Olympic Games is not entirely clear. What we do know is that the Games started as a festival in honour of Zeus, the father of the Greek gods of Mount Olympus. The first recorded Olympics date back to 776 B.C., and the Games were held at regular intervals until A.D. 394, when the Christian Roman Emperor who ruled Greece abolished them because he felt they went against Christian beliefs.

However, the memory of the Games did not die out. In 1636, the English held Olympic Games for English competitors and continued to do so over the next two hundred years. In 1850, an Olympic Society was founded by Dr Penny Brook. Interest in the Olympics was increasing and, at the same time, Britain was developing a sporting tradition in its public schools.

A Frenchman, Baron Pierre de Coubertin, was so impressed by the sportsmanship in the British schools that he decided to set up a modern Olympics based on this sportsmanship and on the ancient Greek Games. Such an Olympics would bring together all the young athletes of the world united in friendly competition, ignoring the divisions of nationality, race and religion. The Baron formed an international committee in 1894 to revive the Games in Greece. Greece, however, was a poor nation at this stage, and it looked as though the attempt would fail. The Crown Prince of Greece stepped in to help. With his help, donations were collected in Greece and from abroad to build sporting facilities for the first modern Olympics.

It was decided that the Olympic Games should be held in the first year of an Olympiad, which is a period of four years. The first year of every Olympiad can be divided by four. The first modern Olympics was held in 1896 in Athens.

## The first Games

King George I of Greece opened the Games, and the Olympic theme was played. This theme has become the official anthem of the Games today.

The first athletes were all men, the majority of whom paid their own expenses. Thirteen countries were represented. Of the 311 athletes who competed, 230 came from Greece itself, 19 were from Germany, 14 from the U.S.A. and 8 from Britain.

The first Olympic winner was the American James Connelly, who won the triple jump. The first three places in the marathon went to Greek athletes, to the delight of the Greek spectators who saw their ancient traditions live again.

The winner of the marathon, Spiros Louis, had gained great physical fitness by running 14 kilometres per day beside his mule which carried water from his village to Athens. When Louis won the marathon, the King offered him a prize of his choice. He asked for a new horse and cart. Other Greeks gave him gifts such as free shaves, hair cuts and meals for life.

Prizes for the athletes of the first Games went only to the first and second place-getters. The winner received a crown of olive branches, a silver medal and a diploma; the second place-getter was awarded a crown of laurel, a bronze medal and a diploma.

The enthusiasm created by the first modern Games led to immediate plans for future Games. Although there were attempts to make Greece the permanent site of the Games, Coubertin pushed through the idea that the Games should be held in a different country each Olympiad.

# Development of the Games

*1900 Paris (France) – IInd Olympiad*
Twenty-two nations were represented; for the first time, women competed, but only in tennis and golf; Charlotte Cooper of Great Britain became the first woman medallist.

*1904 St Louis (U.S.A.) – IIIrd Olympiad*
Twelve nations were represented. Most of the athletes came from the U.S.A. and Canada.

*1908 London (Great Britain) – IVth Olympiad*
Twenty-two countries were represented. The 1908 Games were highly organised and set the administrative pattern for future Olympics. The gold medal for the winner and a winter sport, ice-skating, were introduced. A memorable event was the marathon finish. Pietri, an Italian, led into the stadium. Near collapse, he staggered over the line attended by doctors. He was disqualified, but Queen Alexandria sent him a gold cup as a gesture of admiration.

*1912 Stockholm (Sweden) – Vth Olympiad*
Twenty-eight countries were represented. Women now entered swimming teams.

*1916 Berlin (Germany) – VIth Olympiad*
Cancelled owing to World War I.

*1920 Antwerp (Belgium) – VIIth Olympiad*
Twenty-nine nations competed. Two teenagers, Aileen Riggen (14, U.S.A.) and Nils Skolgun (15, Sweden), won medals in diving.

*1924 Paris (France) – VIIIth Olympiad*
Forty-four nations competed, sending more than 3000 athletes. The first winter games were held in Chamonix, France.

*1928 Amsterdam (Netherlands) – IXth Olympiad*
Forty-eight nations competed. Baron de Coubertin was ill but sent his last message to Olympic athletes asking them "to keep ever alive the flame of the Olympic spirit". Women entered the track and field events. The Olympics had become truly international: Uruguay, Argentina, Chile, India, Japan, Egypt and Haiti, as well as European and North American countries, had gold medallists.

*1932 Los Angeles (U.S.A.) – Xth Olympiad*
Thirty-four nations competed. This Olympics was held during the Great Depression with the world economy in tatters. Many felt it could not be held at all, but the Americans went ahead. Not only did they manage to provide the first Olympic Village, but they also made a profit.

*1936 Berlin (Germany) – XIth Olympiad*
This was the first Olympic Games to be broadcast and televised. It was also the first time that the Olympic torch was lit in Olympia in Greece and transported to the host city to light the Olympic flame. The most outstanding athlete was Jesse Owens, a black American. Hitler, who was in power in Germany, refused to congratulate this great sportsman, who had defeated his rivals, including Germans whom Hitler believed were the "master race".

*1940 Tokyo (Japan)/Helsinki (Finland) – XIIth Olympiad*
The Tokyo Olympic Games were cancelled owing to war in Asia. They were transferred to Helsinki, but were again cancelled owing to World War II.

*1944 London (Great Britain) – XIIIth Olympiad*
Cancelled owing to World War II.

*1948 London (Great Britain) – XIVth Olympiad*
Fifty-nine nations sent approximately 4500 athletes. The Games were becoming massive.

*1952 Helsinki (Finland) – XVth Olympiad*
The U.S.S.R. rejoined the Olympics for the first time since 1912.

*1956 Melbourne (Australia) – XIVth Olympiad*
Australia's first Olympic Games held many problems. Quarantine laws were so strict that equestrian events had to be held in Sweden. In addition, 1956 was the year of the Russian invasion of Hungary, and the Suez crisis in Egypt. The Netherlands withdrew over the Hungarian problem, and the People's Republic of China (communist China) withdrew because the Republic of China, based in

Taiwan, was competing. Spain, Egypt and Lebanon also refused to attend. Nevertheless, 67 countries sent representatives.

The Games were held in November and December for the Australian summer. Britain claimed its first Olympic swimming champion in 32 years through Judy Grinham.

*1960 Rome (Italy) – XVIIth Olympiad*
The Games continued on a massive scale. Boxing saw the emergence of American Cassius Clay who, as Mohammed Ali, was to become one of the greatest professional boxers in the world. These Games were free from political problems, but were spoilt by the death of a Danish cyclist who had used drugs.

*1964 Tokyo (Japan) – XVIIIth Olympiad*
Japan was the first Asian country to host the Games. New records were set – 94 nations took part in a record 163 events.

South Africa had their invitation to the Games withdrawn by the International Olympic Committee (I.O.C.).

Britain's greatest successes came in athletics with Ken Matthews, Lynn Davies, Ann Packer and Mary Rand who all won gold medals.

*1968 Mexico City (Mexico) – XIXth Olympiad*
The holding of the games in Mexico City created the problem of competing at high altitude with its effects on performances. Despite the difficulties experienced by some, many athletes were able to use the conditions to their advantage to break records.

South Africa's invitation to the Games was again withdrawn. Some American black athletes protested at the medal ceremonies against the treatment of black people in America.

Britain's David Hemery won a gold medal in the 400 metres hurdles.

*1972 Munich (West Germany) – XXth Olympiad*
The Munich Olympics are remembered with pride for athletic performances and with great sorrow because of terrorism. Eleven Israelis (athletes and officials) were murdered by terrorists. Nations hosting the games now had to concentrate on security so that such a tragedy might never occur again.

Due to a threatened boycott by many of the African nations Rhodesia's (Zimbabwe) invitation to compete was withdrawn.

The outstanding performances were by swimmers Mark Spitz (U.S.A.) who won seven gold medals and Shane Gould (Australia) who won three gold medals. In gymnastics, Olga Korbut (U.S.S.R.) won five medals: three gold, one silver and one bronze.

*1976 Montreal (Canada) – XXIst Olympiad*
Again, politics played a major role. Many African nations boycotted the Games in protest against apartheid in South Africa and the tour of that country by the New Zealand Rugby team. The cost of staging the Games became an increasing concern. Part of these costs were for the massive security precautions.

*1980 Moscow (U.S.S.R.) – XXIInd Olympiad*
The Moscow Olympics were spectacular, but were also dominated by political problems. The U.S.A. refused to send a team in protest over the Russian military presence in Afghanistan.

British athletes were given a choice – some went, some stayed away. The British athletes Steve Ovett, Sebastian Coe, Alan Wells, and Daley Thompson all won gold medals.

*1984 Los Angeles (U.S.A) – XXIIIth Olympiad*
The Soviet Union and a dozen other nations boycotted the Games. Kristin Otto, a German swimmer, won six gold medals – another record.

*1988 Seoul (South Korea) – XXIVth Olympiad*
The 1988 Seoul Olympic Games were noted for the dramatic disqualification of the 100 metres World Record Holder Ben Johnson (Canada) for drug taking. Tennis appeared for the first time as an Olympic event. Britain's major successes came in the men's hockey and rowing competitions.

*1992 Barcelona (Spain) – XXVth Olympiad*
From 1994 the Winter and Summer Games will be held two years apart, the Winter Games in 1994; the Summer Games in 1996.

**Table 1.1:** British Olympic Medals

| Year | City | Gold | Silver | Bronze | Total |
|---|---|---|---|---|---|
| 1896 | Athens | 3 | 3 | 1 | 7 |
| 1900 | Paris | 17 | 8 | 12 | 37 |
| 1904 | St Louis | 1 | 1 | — | 2 |
| 1906 | Athens | 8 | 11 | 6 | 25 |
| 1908 | London | 57 | 50 | 40 | 147 |
| 1912 | Stockholm | 10 | 15 | 16 | 41 |
| 1920 | Antwerp | 15 | 15 | 13 | 43 |
| 1924 | Paris | 9 | 13 | 12 | 34 |
| 1928 | Amsterdam | 3 | 10 | 7 | 20 |
| 1932 | Los Angeles | 4 | 7 | 5 | 16 |
| 1936 | Berlin | 4 | 7 | 3 | 14 |
| 1948 | London | 3 | 14 | 6 | 23 |
| 1952 | Helsinki | 1 | 2 | 8 | 11 |
| 1956 | Melbourne | 6 | 7 | 11 | 24 |
| 1960 | Rome | 2 | 6 | 12 | 20 |
| 1964 | Tokyo | 4 | 12 | 2 | 18 |
| 1968 | Mexico City | 5 | 5 | 3 | 13 |
| 1972 | Munich | 4 | 5 | 9 | 18 |
| 1976 | Montreal | 3 | 5 | 5 | 13 |
| 1980 | Moscow | 5 | 7 | 9 | 21 |
| 1984 | Los Angeles | 5 | 11 | 21 | 37 |
| 1988 | Seoul | 5 | 10 | 9 | 24 |

## Some great Olympians

Many athletes have excelled in individual events. Some, however, have performed so well over a range of events or over several Olympics that they are outstanding in the history of sport.

*Jim Thorpe*

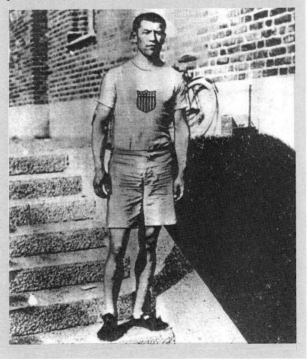

In 1912, the King of Sweden called Jim Thorpe "the greatest athlete in the world". Many still consider him the greatest athlete of the first half of the twentieth century. He is the only person to have won the gold medal in the decathlon and pentathlon in one Olympics. He was stripped of his honours after he was accused of being a professional because he had accepted payment for a month's games of baseball. Only amateurs could compete in the Olympic Games. Recently, many years after his death, he was reinstated on the honour roll of the Olympics. Thorpe, an American, was a descendant of Chief Black Hawk. His early life was tragic – his father, mother and twin brother all died before he was 16. At 16 he was only 1.4 metres tall and weighed only 52 kilograms. Through perseverance and playing football, he built himself up to the stage where he could compete in five Olympic events in one day.

*Paavo Nurmi*

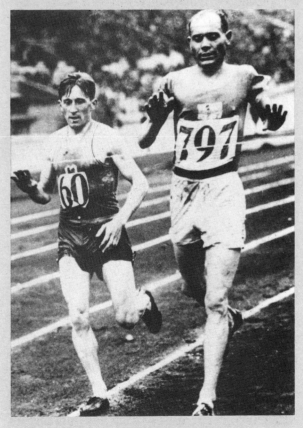

The "Flying Finn", as Paavo Nurmi (right) was called, was considered by many to be the greatest runner of the first half of this century. He was admired particularly for his will and determination. Paavo was the son of a Finnish woodworker. He started running when he was very young though his talent was first recognised when he was called up for his national service in the Finnish army. He had to undertake a 15-kilometre march in full uniform carrying a rifle, cartridge case and back-pack filled with sand. When he was told as a joke that he could run if he wanted to, he took up the challenge and completed the course in less than an hour to the astonishment of all.

At the 1920 Games, he won the 10 000 metres and the cross-country race, but it was at the Paris Games in 1924 that he became a legend. He won the 1500 metres; just one hour later he took the gold for the 5000 metres. Two days later he won the 10 000-metre cross-country. In 1928, he won the 10 000 metres. In 1932, he was to run the marathon, but the International Amateur Federation declared him a professional because of his expense account during a tour of Germany, and he was not allowed to compete.

During his career, he won six gold medals at the Olympics and held world records for the one mile, the 3, 4, 5 and 10 miles, the 3000, 5000, 10 000 and 15 000 metres and for the total distance a person could run in one hour. In 1952, it was Paavo Nurmi who ran into the Helsinki Stadium with the torch to light the Olympic flame. The crowd applauded this great athlete, then 55 years old. Though his records have been broken, Paavo Nurmi remains an example to all athletes for his achievements.

### Johnny Weismuller

Johnny was a hero of the United States in the 1920s. Although sickly as a child, he became the world's fastest swimmer over 100 metres and was recognised as the greatest swimmer in the first half of this century. His fame led Hollywood to offer Johnny the role of Tarzan, and he was often filmed swimming swiftly across alligator-infested rivers to save the legendary Jane.

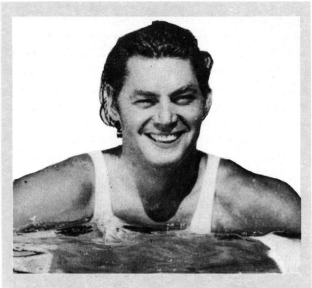

For a long time, Johnny Weismuller held the record for gaining gold medals for the 100 metres in two consecutive Olympics, until Dawn Fraser gained gold in three consecutive Games. His medals were:

- Paris, 1924:

| | |
|---|---|
| 100 m freestyle | gold |
| 400 m freestyle | gold |
| 4 × 200 m freestyle relay | gold |
| water polo | bronze |

- Amsterdam, 1928:

| | |
|---|---|
| 100 m freestyle | gold |
| 4 × 200 m freestyle relay | gold |

### Jesse Owens

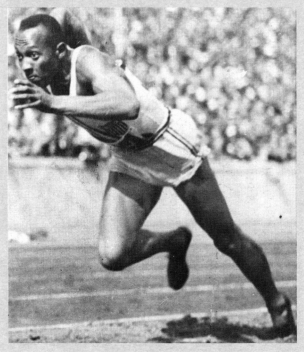

As a young boy of 12, Jesse Owens of the U.S.A. dreamed of winning a gold medal in the Olympics. His performance in the 1936 Berlin Olympics assured him a place in the history of sport. Some consider him the greatest athlete of the first half of this century, greater even than Jim Thorpe. He won track gold medals for the 100 metres, 200 metres and the 4 × 100-metre relay, and also a gold medal for the long jump.

*Dawn Fraser*

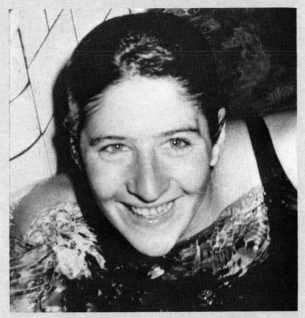

The Australian Dawn Fraser is one of the world's greatest swimmers. As a child, Dawn was unwell, and suffered from asthma and pleurisy. However, Dawn dominated world swimming for over 12 years, winning the 100-metres freestyle in three Olympic Games.

Dawn's swimming achievements are most impressive:

- Melbourne, 1956:

  | | |
  |---|---|
  | 100m freestyle | gold |
  | 4 × 100 m freestyle relay | gold |
  | 400 m freestyle | silver |

- Rome, 1960:

  | | |
  |---|---|
  | 100 m freestyle | gold |
  | 4 × 100 m freestyle relay | silver |
  | 4 × 100 m medley relay | silver |

- Tokyo, 1964:

  | | |
  |---|---|
  | 100 m freestyle | gold |
  | 4 × 100 m freestyle relay | silver |

*Nadia Comaneci*

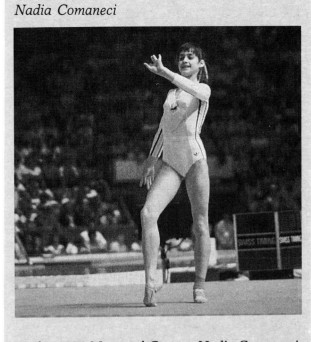

At the 1976 Montreal Games, Nadia Comaneci from Romania was awarded maximum points for her performances on the beam and the asymmetric bars. At the time she was only 14, less than 1.5 metres tall and weighed 39 kilograms. This was the first perfect "10" in gymnastics history, which she repeated at the Moscow Olympics in 1980. Her performances along with those of the Russian gymnast Olga Korbut raised public interest in gymnastics.

*Mark Spitz*

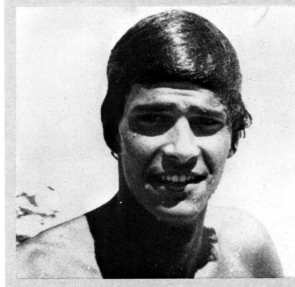

Mark Spitz was called the "human torpedo". Swimming for the United States in the 1972

Olympics, Spitz won seven gold medals in only eight days, all in record time. Although his major stroke was freestyle, he also dominated the butterfly events. On his return to the United States, he was paid enormous fees for advertising products and for coaching swimming. His medals were:

- Mexico City, 1968:

| | |
|---|---|
| 4 × 100 m freestyle relay | gold |
| 4 × 200 m freestyle relay | gold |
| 100 m butterfly | silver |
| 100 m freestyle | bronze |

- Munich, 1972:

| | |
|---|---|
| 4 × 100 m freestyle relay | gold |
| 4 × 200 m freestyle relay | gold |
| 4 × 100 m medley relay | gold |
| 100 m freestyle | gold |
| 200 m freestyle | gold |
| 100 m butterfly | gold |
| 200 m butterfly | gold |

*Carl Lewis*

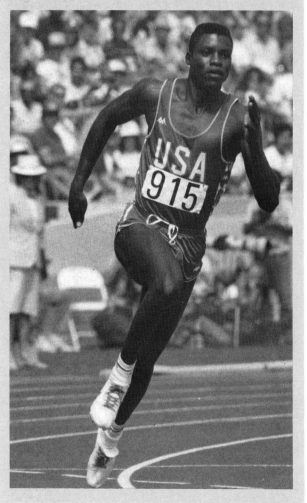

In the 1984 Olympics, Carl Lewis equalled Jesse Owens' 1936 record, taking gold for exactly the same events: 100 metres, 200 metres, 4 × 100 metres relay and the long jump. He is considered one of the world's most outstanding athletes.

*Daley Thompson*

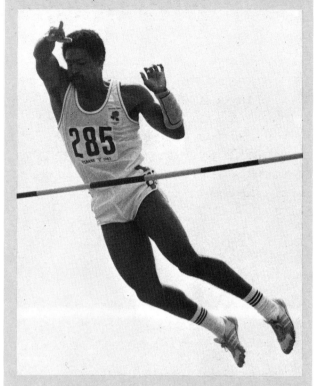

Daley Thompson considered by many to be the world's best all-round athlete at his peak. He won the gold medal for the decathlon in the 1980 and 1984 Olympics, and also in the Commonwealth Games of 1978, 1982 and 1986.

## To the future

In 1973, the Olympic Congress adopted as its motto, "Sport for a world of peace". The hope continues that the ideals behind the modern Olympics will triumph. Despite all the problems, the Olympic Games still foster excellence in human performance. Apart from medal winners, there are many athletes who have displayed the dedication and courage required to compete at Olympic level.

# Unit B

## Foundations of physical education

To improve performance in physical activities, it is necessary to have a basis or foundation of knowledge about the body and its workings, about commonly used methods of improving body movement and about how people interact in sport.

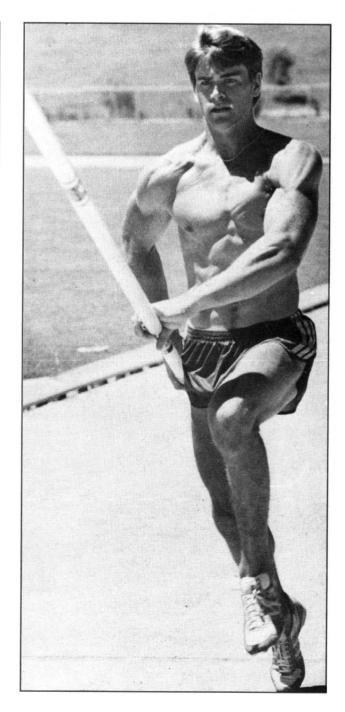

# Your body

In this chapter you will study the human body and how it works. This knowledge is important so that you can understand:
- how your body moves and works most efficiently
- how to care for the body.

## The human body

The human body is a most complex and marvellous organism. Even today we still do not understand all of its secrets. The body is often called a living machine because it consists of many parts, all with different functions. The proper functioning of the body depends on all the different parts working together in harmony.

## What is the body made of?

The human body consists of millions of tiny cells. These cells are not all the same — they are different shapes and sizes, and have different jobs to do. Cells join together to form tissue and various tissues join together to form organs. Organs work together in systems which perform many of the functions of the body (see figure 2.1).

## Systems of the body

There are ten body systems:
- Skeletal system
- Muscular system
- Circulatory system
- Respiratory system
- Digestive system
- Excretory system
- Reproductive system
- Nervous system
- Endocrine system
- Skin system

**Table 2.1:** The body systems and their functions

| System | Main organ | Main function |
|---|---|---|
| Skeletal | — | Provides a rigid framework which supports the body |
| Muscular | — | Provides movement |
| Circulatory | Heart | Transports blood |
| Respiratory | Lungs | Oxygenates the blood; disposes of carbon dioxide |
| Digestive | Stomach; intestines | Digests food |
| Excretory | Kidneys | Removes waste products |
| Reproductive | Sexual organs | Reproduces |
| Nervous | Brain | Controls all the body systems |
| Endocrine | Pituitary gland | Releases hormones which aid the nervous system in controlling the body |
| Skin | Skin | Provides protection and temperature control |

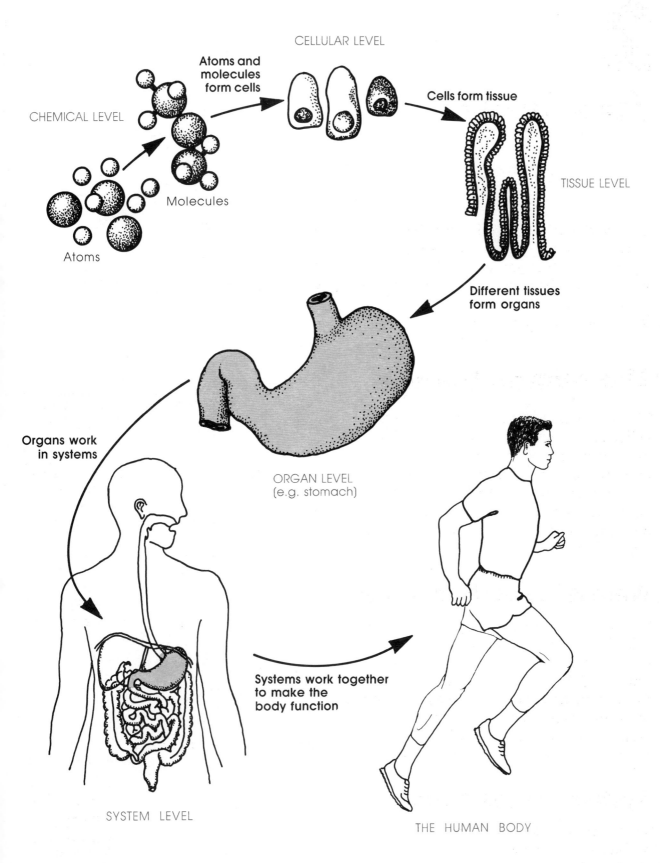

**Figure 2.1:** Cells join together to form tissue. Different tissues join together to form an organ and organs work together to form systems.

# The skeletal system

All the bones of the body (more than two hundred) form the skeletal system.

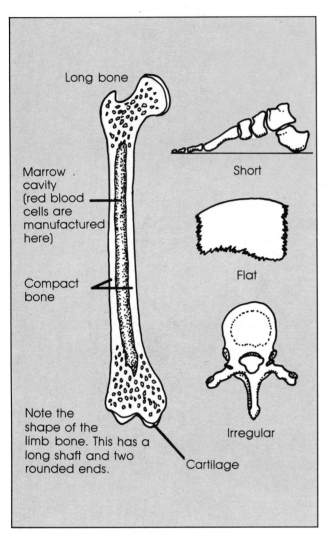

**Figure 2.2:** Types of bones.

# The functions of the skeletal system

The skeletal system:
- provides the rigid framework of the body, giving shape to the body
- provides support for muscles
- protects vital and delicate internal organs such as the brain, heart, lungs and liver
- manufactures blood cells
- stores mineral salts especially calcium.

# The structure and workings of the skeletal system

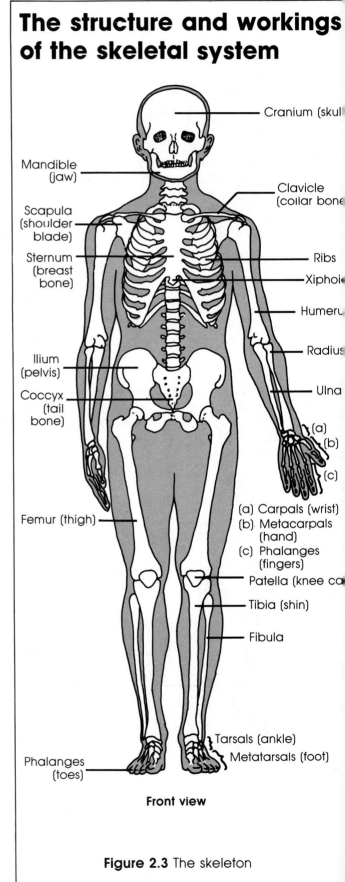

**Figure 2.3** The skeleton

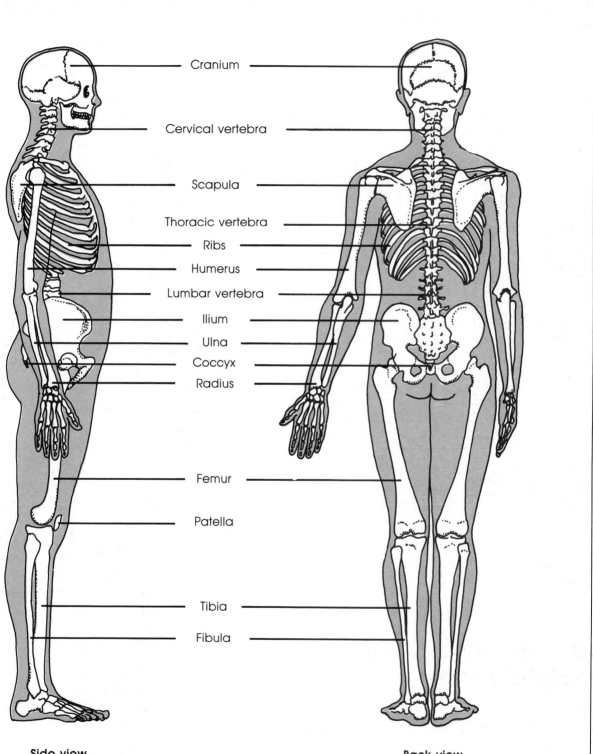

Cranium

Cervical vertebra

Scapula

Thoracic vertebra

Ribs

Humerus

Lumbar vertebra

Ilium

Ulna

Coccyx

Radius

Femur

Patella

Tibia

Fibula

**Side view**

**Back view**

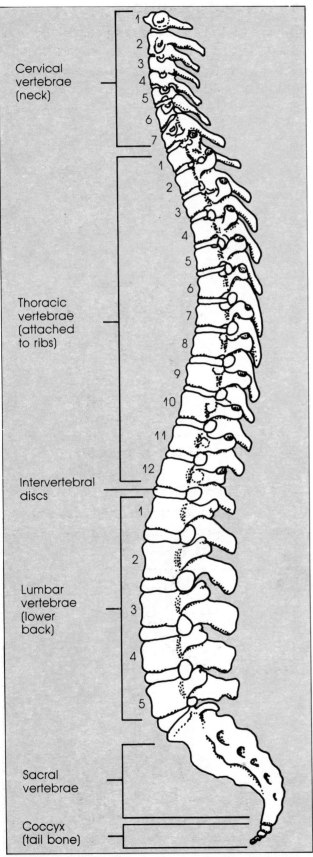

Cervical vertebrae (neck)

1
2
3
4
5
6
7

Thoracic vertebrae (attached to ribs)

1
2
3
4
5
6
7
8
9
10
11
12

Intervertebral discs

Lumbar vertebrae (lower back)

1
2
3
4
5

Sacral vertebrae

Coccyx (tail bone)

**Figure 2.4:** The vertebral column (spine) keeps the body upright, protects the spinal cord and helps in posture and movement.

# Development of the skeleton

The skeleton is formed during the first three months of foetal existence. At first it is made from cartilage tissue (the type of tissue forming the hard part of your nose). When a child is born, the skeleton has not yet hardened. The hardening occurs gradually. To harden into mature and strong bones, the skeleton needs calcium. The skeleton continues to grow in length until about the age of 13–15 in girls and 16–18 in boys.

# Joints

## What are joints?

Joints are the areas where two or more bones meet. There are three types of joints:

● *Fixed or immoveable joints* such as those in the skull.

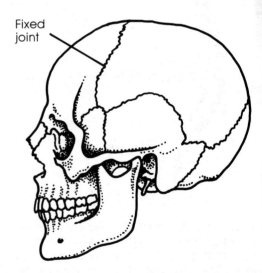

Fixed joint

**Figure 2.5:** A fixed joint (skull).

● *Slightly moveable joints.* These joints allow for only a small amount of movement. One example is found where the ribs join the breastbone; another is the vertebrae of the spine. These joints are sometimes called cartilaginous joints because cartilage separates the adjoining bones.

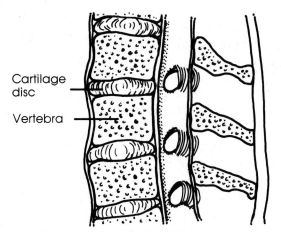

**Figure 2.6:** A slightly moveable joint (spine).

- *Freely moveable joints, often called synovial joints.* These are the most common of the three types of joints. These joints allow movement in one or more directions. They are lubricated by synovial fluid.

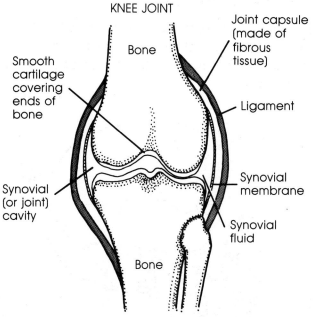

**Figure 2.7:** The structure of a typical synovial joint. *Ligaments* are tough, fibrous cords attached to the bones. They bind and strengthen the capsule, thus helping to join the bones.

## Types of freely moveable joints

There are several types of freely moveable joints:

- ball and socket
- hinge
- pivot
- condyloid
- gliding
- saddle.

## The ball and socket joint

This joint allows a wide range of movement which is made possible by a round-headed bone fitting into a cup-shaped socket. The hip and shoulder joints are examples.

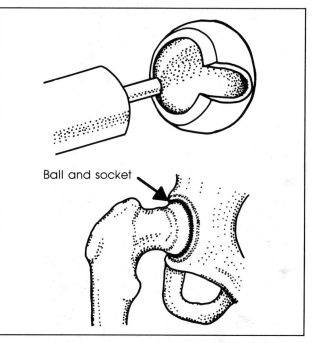

**Figure 2.8:** The ball and socket joint.

## The hinge joint

The hinge joint allows movement in only one direction. Hinge joints are found in the elbow, knee and ankle.

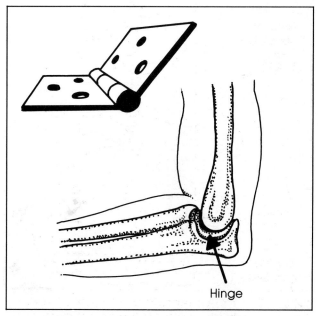

**Figure 2.9:** The hinge joint.

## The pivot joint

This joint allows a rotation movement. Examples are the joint which allows us to turn our heads from side to side and the joint which allows us to turn our hands over and back.

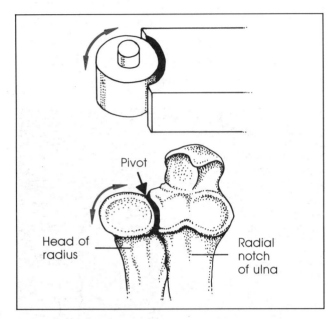

**Figure 2.10:** The pivot joint.

## The condyloid joint

The condyloid joint is basically a hinge joint which also allows some sidewards movement. Such a joint allows wrist movement.

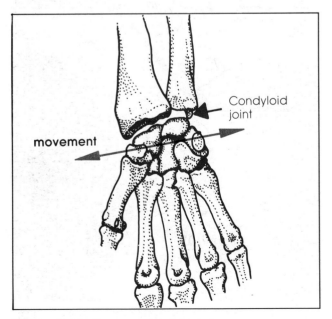

**Figure 2.11:** The condyloid joint.

## The gliding joint

The gliding joint allows gliding between two flat surfaces. Such joints are found between the small bones of the wrist.

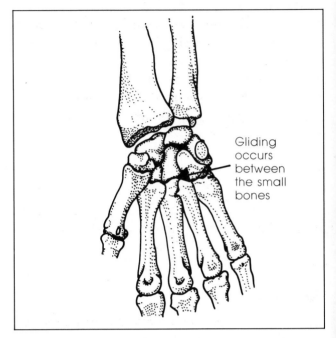

**Figure 2.12:** The gliding joint.

## The saddle joint

The saddle joint allows a free hinge-like movement in two directions. Such a joint gives the thumb its movement, allowing the hand to accomplish delicate tasks.

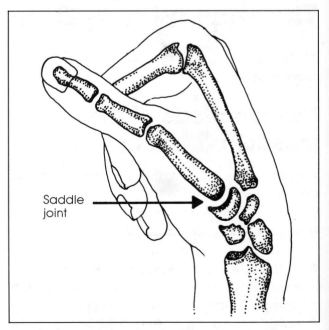

**Figure 2.13:** The saddle joint.

# Connective tissue

Connective tissue exists in many forms throughout the body. It does many jobs including:

- supporting and nourishing other tissue;
- providing packing material between organs;
- helping in movement.

During physical activity, the most important connective tissues are cartilage, ligaments and tendons.

## Cartilage

Cartilage is a glassy, smooth tissue. It is found in various forms in the body. Examples are the hard part of the ear and the cartilage found between the bones of the vertebral column.

## Ligaments

Ligaments are bands of elastic fibrous tissue. They link bones together.

## Tendons

Tendons are strong, non-elastic cords that join muscles to bones and, therefore, allow movement to take place.

# The muscular system

All the muscles of the body form the muscular system.

## The functions of the muscular system

Through its many muscles, the muscular system:

- allows human movement
- allows the development of strength, endurance and speed
- helps other body systems do their work. Examples are the heart muscle, which pumps blood around the body, and the muscles in the chest, which aid in breathing.

# The structure and workings of the muscular system

There are more than six hundred muscles of the body, all with special jobs. The nervous system controls the action of the muscles, and the circulatory system supplies the muscles with a rich blood supply, which provides fuel for the muscles.

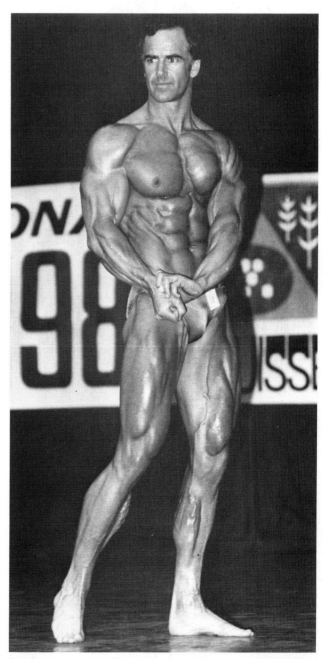

There are more than six hundred muscles in the body, and each has a special job.

# Types of muscles

There are three types of muscle:
- Striated or skeletal muscles are attached to the skeleton. These muscles are controlled consciously when the person decides to move, so they are often called *voluntary muscles.*

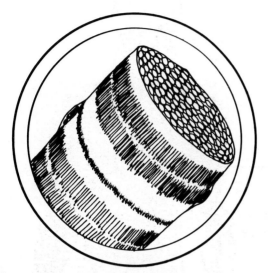

**Figure 2.14:** Striated or striped muscle looks like bundles of fibre held together by other tissue. The mass of fibres group together to form an elliptical body called a belly.

- Smooth muscles are mostly found in layers and form the muscle part of the digestive tract, the bladder, blood vessels and the skin. They are not controlled consciously, so are often called *involuntary muscles.*

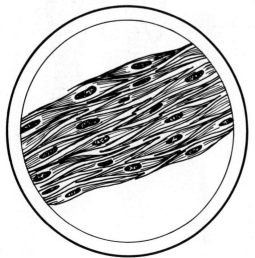

**Figure 2.15:** A smooth muscle, often called an involuntary muscle.

- Cardiac muscle forms the major part of the heart, and contracts and relaxes continuously to provide the pumping action. This action is not consciously controlled, so cardiac muscle is also *involuntary muscle.*

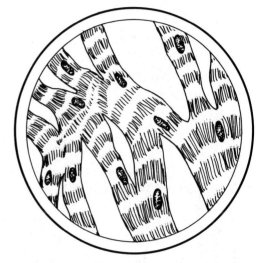

**Figure 2.16:** Cardiac muscle.

# Skeletal muscles and movement

## Attachment to the bones

Skeletal muscles are attached to bones usually by tendons. The attachment of the tendon of a muscle which moves the bone is called the insertion of the muscle. The attachment of the tendon which acts as an anchor point is called the origin.

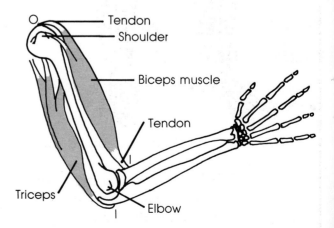
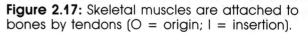

**Figure 2.17:** Skeletal muscles are attached to bones by tendons (O = origin; I = insertion).

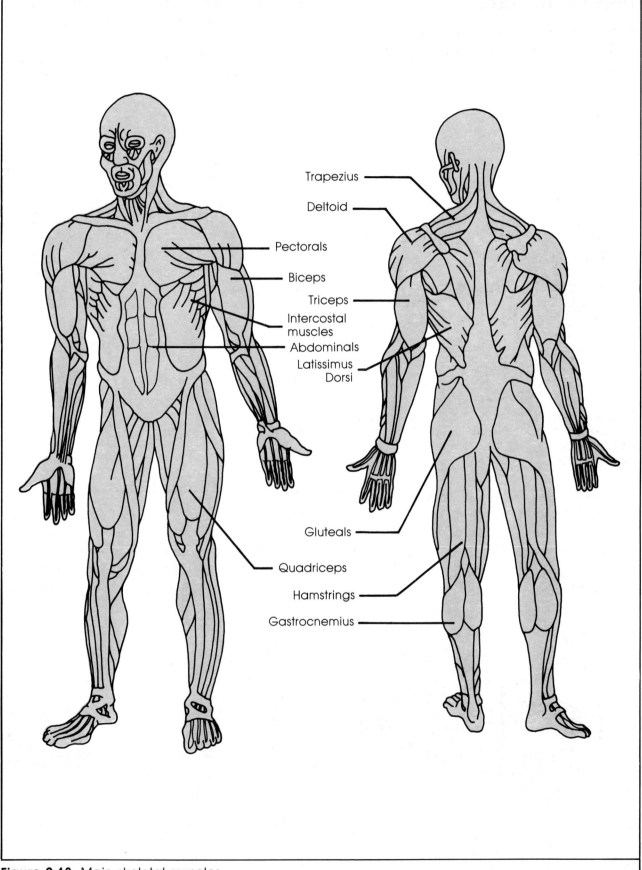

**Figure 2.18:** Main skeletal muscles.

## The muscles at work

When you move a part of your body, some muscles must contract. Muscles shorten and bulge when contracted; they return to their original length when relaxed. There are two main types of muscle contraction:

- Isotonic contractions occur when any part of the body moves, and involves a change in the length of the muscles. There are two types of isotonic contractions:
  - *Concentric contraction* occurs when the muscle shortens, for example when you bend your arm upwards;

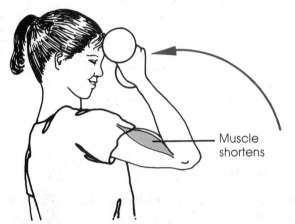

Muscle shortens

**Figure 2.19:** Concentric contraction.

- *Eccentric contraction* occurs when there is a gradual controlled release of a muscle contraction. This is often called a "lengthening" contraction, although the word "lengthening" is misleading. In fact, most muscles do not actually lengthen; they merely return to their normal resting length.

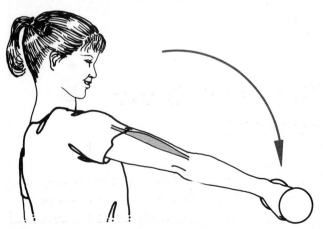

**Figure 2.20:** Eccentric contraction.

- Isometric contractions do not change the length of the muscle and do not cause movement. Examples of isometric muscle contractions are pushing against a wall or holding an object in a stationary position.

To allow movement, muscles work in pairs. For example, when you bend your arms upwards, the muscle of the upper arm contracts while other muscles relax. The muscles which contract to carry out the movement are called *prime movers*. The muscles which relax to allow this movement are called *antagonists*.

Muscles at work are given different names according to the role they play in movement. Examples are:

- Flexors – muscles that bend a limb at a joint.

- Extensors – muscles that straighten a limb at a joint.

- Adductors – muscles that move limbs towards the midline of the body.

- Abductors – muscles that move limbs away from the midline of the body.

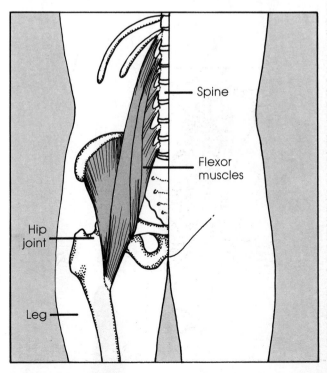

Spine

Flexor muscles

Hip joint

Leg

**Figure 2.21:** These flexor muscles of the hip joint allow the thigh to be raised.

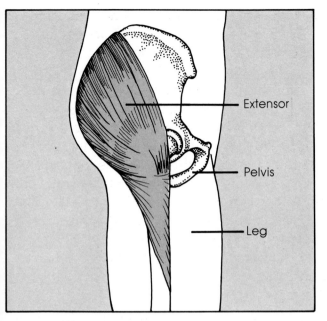

**Figure 2.22:** This extensor of the hip joint allows the thigh to be straightened.

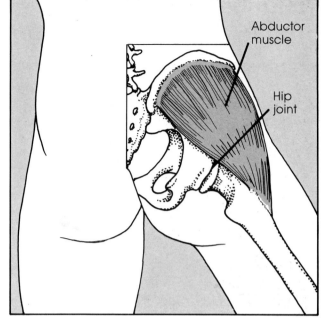

**Figure 2.24:** These abductor muscles of the hip joint allow the legs to be parted.

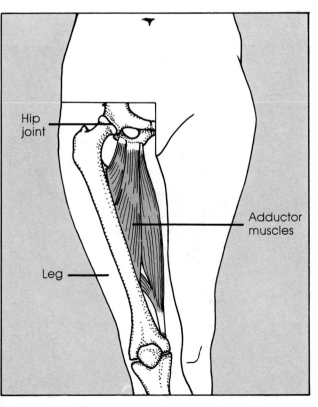

**Figure 2.23:** These adductor muscles of the hip joint allow the knees to be brought together.

## Muscle tone

Muscle tone is the tension of the muscular system. It can be described as the state of readiness of the muscular system to do its job. Muscle tone is not constant. It decreases in times of relaxation and increases dramatically in states of excitement such as fear, anger or stress. Muscle tone is extremely important. Poor muscle tone leads to posture defects, loss of strength and loss of muscle endurance, and makes recovery from disease or injury harder. Exercise increases muscle tone.

# The circulatory system

The circulatory system is the transport system by which blood is carried to all parts of the body. All other body systems depend on its functioning efficiently.

# The functions of the circulatory system

The circulatory system:

- circulates blood through the body
- transports water, oxygen and food to cells and removes wastes from the cells
- helps other body systems to function; for example, blood supply to muscles is increased during exercise
- helps fight disease
- helps maintain correct body temperature.

# The structure and workings of the circulatory system

The circulatory system has three parts:

- The heart – the organ which pumps blood around the body.
- The blood vessels – the tubes (arteries, capillaries and veins) through which the blood moves.
- The blood itself. The average adult has about 5 litres of blood.

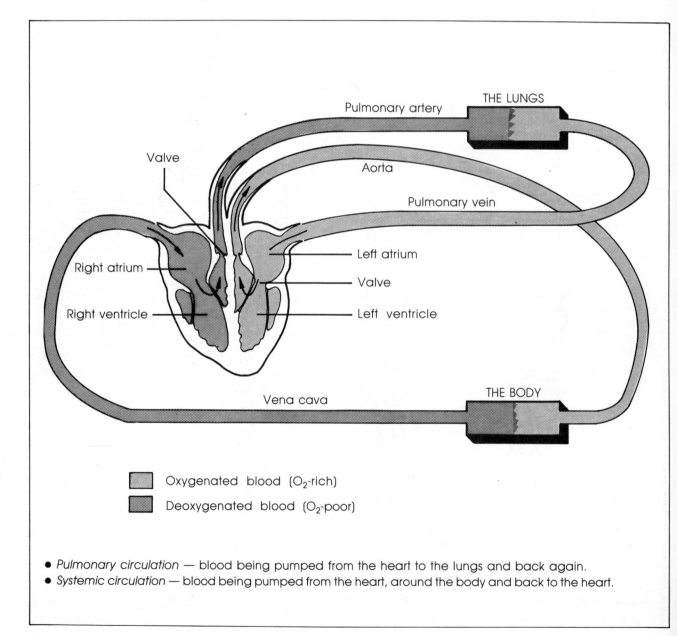

- *Pulmonary circulation* — blood being pumped from the heart to the lungs and back again.
- *Systemic circulation* — blood being pumped from the heart, around the body and back to the heart.

**Figure 2.25:** Diagrammatic view of the heart and the circulatory system.

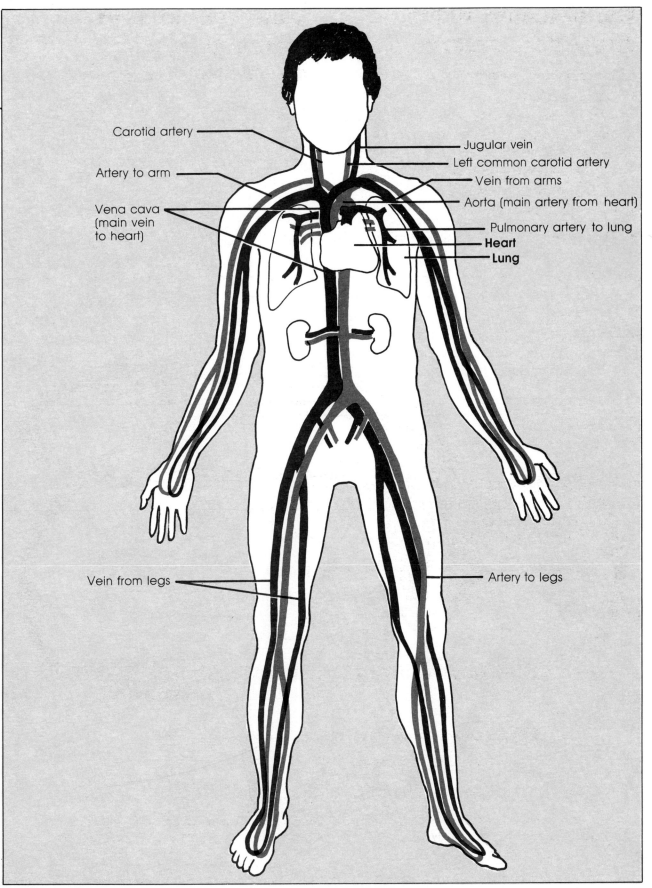

Carotid artery

Artery to arm

Vena cava
(main vein
to heart)

Jugular vein

Left common carotid artery

Vein from arms

Aorta (main artery from heart)

Pulmonary artery to lung

**Heart**

**Lung**

Vein from legs

Artery to legs

**Figure 2.26:** The circulatory system.

# The heart

The heart itself is a hollow, muscular organ which serves as a pump to push blood around the body. It is located in the centre of the chest between the two lungs and behind the protection of the ribs. The lower portion extends to the left of the chest. It is about the size of two average adult fists. The heart is capable of pumping blood about two metres into the air if a large artery is cut. The heart is divided into four chambers. A muscular wall divides it into the right and left sides. Each side consists of two chambers: the upper chamber is called the atrium, and the lower chamber is the ventricle. Blood flows into the atrium, which pushes the blood through a valve into the ventricle. This valve ensures that blood does not flow back into the atrium.

The right-hand side of the heart receives blood in its atrium from the veins. This blood is dark red because its oxygen has been used up. The right atrium pumps this blood into the right ventricle, which in turn pumps the blood through an artery into the lungs where the blood regains oxygen and becomes bright red in colour. From the lungs, the blood flows to the left atrium through a large vein. The left atrium pumps the blood into the left ventricle. The left ventricle is the most powerful part of the heart and pushes the blood through the aorta to the rest of the body.

The average adult heart beats around 72 times per minute when the body is at rest. This circulates the 5 litres of blood in about one minute. However, the number of beats depends on many factors, such as a person's fitness or health, the amount of physical activity and the emotional state of the person.

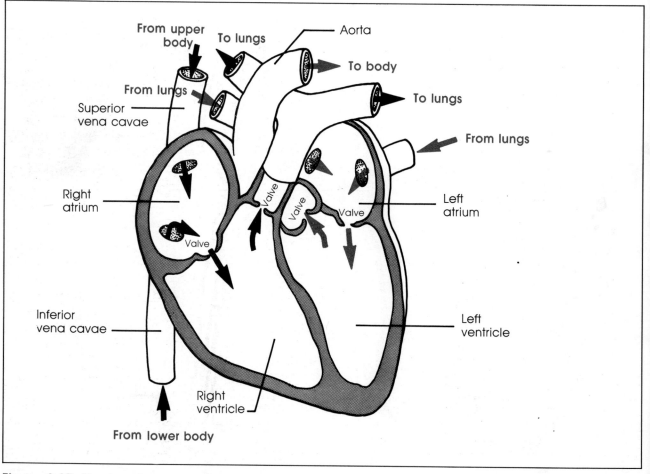

**Figure 2.27:** The heart.

## The pulse

The heartbeat can be counted through the pulse which can be felt and sometimes seen in the arteries just below the skin in certain parts of the body. The pulse occurs when the left ventricle contracts and forces blood into the aorta. The new blood pushes blood already there further on. This movement of the blood in the artery system can be felt as the pulse. The pulse is normally checked on the radial artery on the inside of the wrist. Another popular place is on the carotid artery in the neck. Under normal situations, for a healthy adult, the pulse will be regular and strong.

## The blood vessels

There are three main types of blood vessels:
● arteries
● capillaries
● veins.

### Arteries

Arteries, whose job it is to carry blood *from the heart* to the rest of the body, are the thickest of the blood vessels. The aorta is the largest artery of the body and carries blood straight from the heart; the smallest arteries, called arterioles, carry the blood to the capillaries. Blood in arteries is bright red owing to the presence of oxygen. The exception is the artery leading to the lungs.

### Capillaries

Arteries ⟶ Veins
via Capillaries

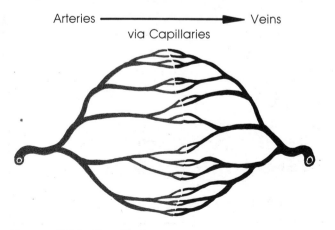

**Figure 2.28:** Capillaries.

There are more than 100 000 kilometres of capillaries in the body which form a vast network through the body tissue. Capillaries are very thin blood vessels, thinner even than human hair, and most let only single cells of blood through one after another. Through the walls of the capillaries, oxygen and nutrients are passed into cells and carbon dioxide and waste products are taken away. At the end of the capillaries, blood flows into the veins.

## Veins

Veins have thinner walls than arteries. Their job is to take blood back to the heart. They contain valves to prevent the blood flowing backwards. The blood in veins is dark red, indicating the presence of carbon dioxide and less oxygen. The exception is the vein carrying blood from the lungs to the heart.

## Blood pressure

Blood pressure is the pressure exerted by blood on the walls of the blood vessels. However, when we talk about a person's "blood pressure", we refer to the measurement of blood pressure in the large artery found above the elbow. This measurement is expressed in two ways.

● Systolic pressure is measured when the left ventricle of the heart contracts.
● Diastolic pressure is measured when the left ventricle of the heart is relaxed.

Blood pressure is expressed as a fraction:

$$\frac{\text{systolic pressure}}{\text{diastolic pressure}}$$

Average blood pressure is $\frac{120}{80}$ (the measurements are millimetres of mercury). The normal range for healthy adults at rest is between $\frac{100}{60}$ and $\frac{140}{90}$.

**Table 2.2:** Average arterial blood pressures at different ages (mm Hg)

| Age | Systolic | Diastolic |
|---|---|---|
| Newborn | 40 | 20 |
| 1 month | 75 | 50 |
| 2 years | 85 | 60 |
| 4 years | 90 | 65 |
| 10 years | 105 | 70 |
| 15 years | 110 | 70 |
| 20 years | 120 | 80 |
| 30 years | 130 | 85 |
| 40 years | 140 | 90 |
| 50 years | 145 | 90 |
| 60 years | 150 | 90 |

*Source:* William F. Evans, *Anatomy and Physiology,* 2nd ed. (Englewood Cliffs: Prentice Hall, 1971), p. 276.

Blood pressure normally depends on:
- the strength and rate of the heart's contraction;
- the elasticity of blood vessels;
- the amount of blood in the system.

However, a person who becomes afraid, excited, worried or nervous will have an increase in blood pressure, but this will usually be temporary. Consistent high blood pressure is usually a sign of a health problem.

## Blood

Blood makes up about 7 per cent of body weight. Blood is composed of:
- Plasma. About 55 per cent of blood is plasma which is mainly water. Plasma also contains proteins, salts, glucose, fats, antibodies, waste products and some oxygen and carbon dioxide.
- Cells. About 45 per cent of blood is solid material made up of different cells:
  - *Red blood cells (erythrocytes).* These are very tiny and millions would fit on a pin head. Haemoglobin is found in these cells and is responsible for carrying oxygen and carbon dioxide. Haemoglobin carrying oxygen is bright red, showing that the blood is oxygenated; haemoglobin carrying carbon dioxide is dark red, showing that the blood is deoxygenated.
  - *White blood cells (leucocytes).* There are different types of white blood cells. These colourless cells are not as numerous as the red blood cells. Their main job is to engulf and destroy foreign particles or harmful bacteria which get into tissue or blood. When fighting infection, many white cells are killed. This forms pus in wounds.
- Platelets. Platelets are tiny fragments of large cells. Their job is to help clot blood so that dangerous bleeding cannot occur. They not only help to clot blood if the skin is cut, but they also seal holes and tears in small blood vessels.

## Blood groups

People do not have exactly the same blood composition. There are four main blood groups:
- O (about 45 per cent of people)
- A (about 41 per cent of people)
- B (about 10 per cent of people)
- AB (about 4 per cent of people).

Blood is also categorised by the presence of a special protein. Those who have this protein in the blood are said to be Rh-positive (Rh+). Those without it are said to be Rh-negative (Rh−). Even when people have the same blood group, their blood may not match exactly.

# The respiratory system

The respiratory system is the body's breathing system.

# The functions of the respiratory system

The respiratory system:
- brings oxygen from the atmosphere into the lungs

- provides, inside the lungs, a method of gas exchange that allows oxygen to enter the blood and carbon dioxide to leave the blood
- removes carbon dioxide and some water vapour from the lungs into the atmosphere.

As well, the movement of air from the lungs through the vocal cords enables a person to speak.

# The structure and workings of the respiratory system

The respiratory system consists of:
- Air passages
- Lungs
- Diaphragm

## Air passages

### The nasal cavity

The nostrils form the entrance to the nasal cavity. Small hairs called cilia found in the nostrils filter out dust, pollen and other impurities. The nasal cavity warms and moistens air to assist it on its journey to the lungs.

### The pharynx

The pharynx allows the passage of air and food. Food is swallowed into the oesophagus and the air passes into the larynx.

### The larynx

The larynx is often called the "voice box". Air passes through the larynx into the trachea. At the upper opening of the larynx is the epiglottis, which automatically prevents food from entering the larynx and getting

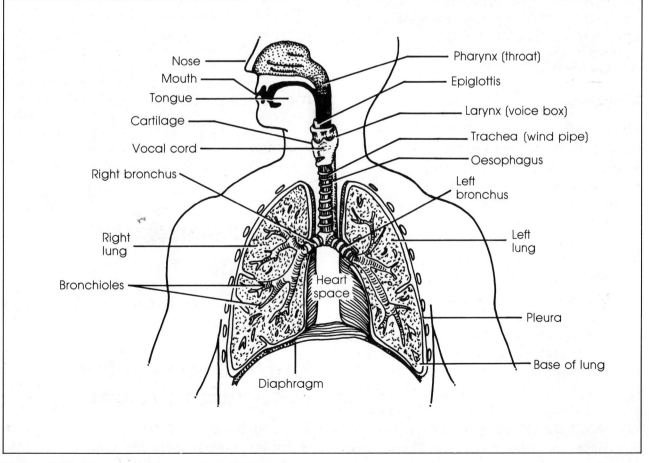

**Figure 2.29:** The respiratory system.

into the lungs. Inside the larynx are the vocal cords which allow voice production.

### The trachea

The trachea is the windpipe through which air passes to the bronchi. It must remain open or the whole respiratory system fails. The trachea consists of strong cartilage rings ensuring that it is always kept open.

### The bronchi

The trachea branches into two bronchi, one for each lung. Each of the bronchi divide into smaller and smaller branches called *bronchioles.* These tiny structures end in millions of microscopic air sacs called *alveoli.* Each of these is surrounded by capillaries and this is where the exchange of oxygen for carbon dioxide takes place.

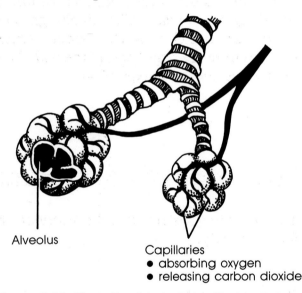

Alveolus

Capillaries
● absorbing oxygen
● releasing carbon dioxide

**Figure 2.30:** The alveolus and capillaries.

### The lungs

The lungs are the major organs of the respiratory system and take up most of the chest cavity. The lungs look and feel spongy because of the many tiny bronchioles and the millions of air sacs. The lungs are covered by membrane called the pleura. Pleura also lines the inside of the chest and the top of the diaphragm. Pleura is smooth and moist to prevent friction as the lungs expand and contract in breathing.

### The diaphragm

The diaphragm is a muscle found below the lungs sealing off the chest from the abdominal cavity. As the lungs have no muscles of their own, their expansion and contraction depends on the movement of the diaphragm. Thus it is the diaphragm, not the lungs, which is responsible for the process of breathing.

# Breathing

Renewal of air in the lungs is caused by two types of breathing:
● inspiration – breathing in
● expiration – breathing out.

Breathing is automatically controlled by the brain. The brain monitors the level of carbon dioxide in the blood. It is the growing level of carbon dioxide which makes the brain signal the diaphragm to move, causing the breathing in of oxygen in the air.

In adult men, breathing occurs 12–18 times every minute; women breathe slightly faster. When a person is at rest, breathing is slower and shallower than when a person is active or excited.

### Inspiration

The chest cavity is fully enclosed and during breathing it alters its shape and size.

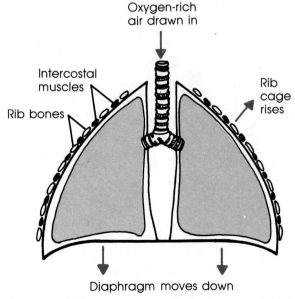

Oxygen-rich
air drawn in

Intercostal
muscles

Rib bones

Rib
cage
rises

Diaphragm moves down

**Figure 2.31:** Inspiration.

When at rest, the diaphragm is shaped like a dome with the upper part of the dome towards the lungs. During inspiration, the diaphragm contracts. The diaphragm flattens and moves downwards. When the diaphragm flattens, the intercostal muscles move the ribs upwards and outwards, further expanding the chest cavity. This expansion decreases the air pressure in the chest cavity, forcing air into the lungs.

- Yawns are extended inspiration.
- Hiccups (hiccoughs) are noisy inspirations. The muscle of the diaphragm goes into irregular spasms causing a sudden sucking-in of air. The air passing through the vocal cords causes the sound.

## Expiration

During expiration, the chest cavity returns to its "at rest" size and shape. The diaphragm relaxes and returns to its dome shape and the ribs return to their original position, increasing the pressure in the chest cavity and so forcing the lungs to expel air.

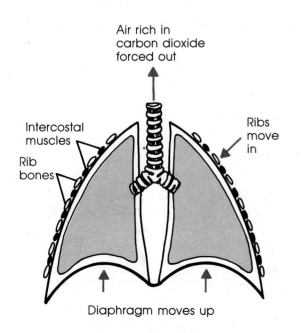

**Figure 2.32:** Expiration.

Coughing is forced expiration. The air is forced quickly through the vocal cords causing the noise. Coughing can help clear the lungs and the bronchi of congestion. However, expired air has water vapour which may contain bacteria. The droplets of water expelled from the respiratory system by coughing are therefore capable of spreading infection.

Normally, when the adult is breathing quietly, about 500 millilitres of air is breathed in and out. However, at some stages, people need more oxygen quickly. This is especially true during physical activity. To increase the chest capacity and therefore increase the amount of air being moved in and out of the lungs, active forced breathing takes place. The diaphragm and intercostal muscles work harder. Other muscles from the upper part of the body help to give greater chest expansion.

# The digestive system

The digestive system absorbs nutrients to feed the body.

## The functions of the digestive system

The digestive system has to perform four processes:
- ingestion – taking in food
- digestion – breaking food down into simpler forms
- absorption – passing the broken-down food into the blood system to feed the body
- excretion – passing wastes from the body.

# The structure and workings of the digestive system

The digestive system consists of:
- the mouth
- the pharynx
- the oesophagus
- the stomach
- the intestines.

This is often called the digestive tract or the alimentary canal. The mouth, the pharynx and the oesophagus are called the upper digestive tract.

These are helped in their work by salivary glands, the liver, the pancreas and the gall bladder.

## Ingestion

### The mouth

Food enters the mouth, where it is moistened by saliva and chewed with the teeth.

---

## Taste

Most tastebuds are found on the tongue, but there are also some on the roof of the mouth and on the pharynx. The tastebuds distinguish:
- sweetness
- saltiness
- sourness
- bitterness.

The sense of taste works well only when the sense of smell is working properly. Most people cannot taste things properly if their nose is blocked off.

---

### The pharynx

From the mouth, food passes with the help of the tongue into the pharynx. From the pharynx it enters the oesophagus. The epiglottis closes off the larynx to ensure food goes towards the stomach and not to the lungs.

### The oesophagus

The oesophagus is commonly called the gullet. It is about 25 centimetres long and ends in the stomach. Muscles force the food down the oesophagus into the stomach. At the end of the oesophagus, a muscle helps prevent food returning from the stomach to the oesophagus.

## Digestion

### The stomach

Although digestion begins in the mouth when saliva acts upon the food, the major part of digestion takes place in the stomach. The stomach receives the food from the upper digestive tract. Involuntary muscles help the stomach mix the food with gastric juices. Gastric juices soften the food and begin to digest it. The food then becomes a creamy liquid called chyme. The stomach wall can also absorb foods such as alcohol, sugar and water.

### The small intestine

The small intestine is narrow but about 6 metres long. It continues the chemical digestion of food already started in the stomach and also absorbs digested food into the blood. The small intestine is divided into three parts: the duodenum, the jejunum and the ileum.

The duodenum's walls produce a digestive juice to finish the breakdown of the food. The pancreas, liver and the gall bladder send juices to help the duodenum's work. The jejunum and ileum have digestive juices as well, but their main job is to absorb the digested food through their walls into the blood which transports the food to the cells.

### The large intestine

After the absorption of food in the small intestine, the fluid waste remaining is passed into the first part of the large intestine, the colon. Here, water and some salts are removed from the fluid waste and enter the

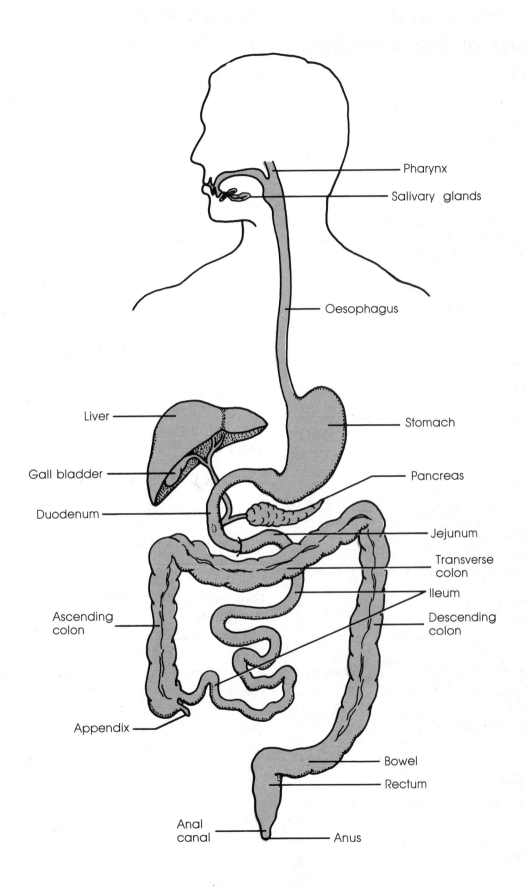

**Figure 2.33:** The digestive system.

blood. The remaining solid waste (faeces) is stored in the last section of the colon, the rectum. It is later passed from the body through the anal canal.

## Organs which aid digestion

### The liver

The liver is the largest organ of the body weighing on average 1.4 kilograms. It receives both oxygenated and deoxygenated blood. The liver:

- produces bile to help digestion
- stores digested food which can be used to provide energy
- stores vitamins
- removes waste products.

### The pancreas

The pancreas is a 15-centimetre-long gland which, as one of its functions, produces juices for digestion.

### The gall bladder

The gall bladder stores bile which passes to the duodenum to break down fats.

# The excretory system

The excretory system is the waste disposal system of the body.

# The functions of the excretory system

The excretory system:

- filters and eliminates waste
- regulates the water content of the body
- regulates the salts of the body.

# The structure and workings of the excretory system

The body excretes through four systems:

- The digestive system, which removes wastes through the bowel.
- The respiratory system, which removes carbon dioxide from the lungs.
- The skin system, which removes water and other wastes through the skin.
- The urinary system, which excretes urine.

# The urinary system

The urinary system consists of:

- the kidneys
- the ureters
- the bladder
- the urethra.

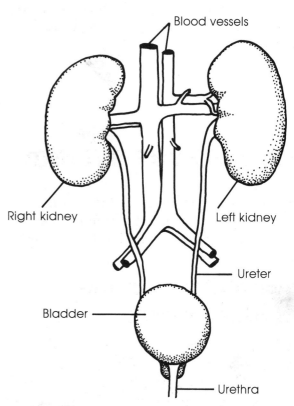

**Figure 2.34:** The urinary system.

After oxygen, water is the second most important need of the body. Water makes up more than half the body weight and accounts for about 90 per cent of blood plasma. An average adult takes in about 1.7 litres of fluid each day to keep the body's 45 litres of water constant. The kidneys control the amount of fluid in the body. Kidneys are dark-red, bean-shaped organs, weighing about 150 grams. Each day about 2000 litres of blood passes through the kidneys.

Inside the kidneys are millions of tiny nephrons which filter the blood. The kidneys remove excess water, drugs, toxins and waste products such as urea, which together form urine.

Normally, only about 1.5 litres of urine are excreted per day, though amounts vary. On hot days, when fluid is being excreted in greater quantities through the skin, the kidneys excrete less urine.

After the kidneys have produced urine, it is passed through tubes called the ureters to the bladder which is a muscular sac acting as a storage tank for the urine. The urine passes out of the body from the bladder through the urethra.

# The nervous system

The nervous system is a most important system as it controls the whole body. It works closely with the endocrine system.

## The functions of the nervous system

The nervous system:
- controls and coordinates the body through a vast network of nerves which act as a communications system
- allows awareness of the body and provides the ability to think and act
- allows awareness of emotion, sensation, memory and of surroundings.

# Structure and workings of the nervous system

Even today we do not fully understand the secrets of the nervous system. However, we do understand a great deal about its workings.

## The neuron

The basic cell of the nervous system is the neuron or nerve cell. When a child is born it has a set number of neurons, more than 10 million in the brain alone. No more neurons are manufactured by the body, so as neurons die they cannot be replaced. Neurons can be destroyed by the ageing process, by oxygen deprivation, through an accident, and by drugs such as alcohol.

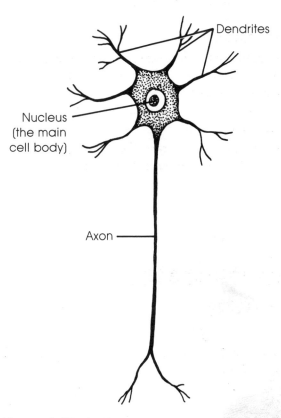

**Figure 2.35:** A neuron.

Neurons come in all shapes and sizes. All neurons have three parts:
- nucleus – the main cell body
- dendrites – fibres which receive impulses and carry them towards the

main cell body; each neuron has about a dozen dendrites

- axons – fibres which transmit impulses away from the main cell body.

The bundles of neuron fibres are called nerves. The fibres are often very long, some exceeding 60 centimetres, and are protected by an insulating sheath.

## Transmission of messages

Axons from one neuron do not join on to dendrites of another neuron. There is always a tiny gap, called a synapse, between them.

Messages have to cross this gap if they are to move on. Thus, a signal travels as an electrical impulse along an axon to its tip where it causes the release of chemicals. These chemicals carry the message across the synapse to a dendrite of the next neuron. The signal then continues as an electrical impulse along this neuron. This process continues until the message reaches its destination. In this way, neurons form a communications network throughout the body. Not all nerves carry messages at the same speed. Some can carry messages at over 500 kilometres per hour; some messages travel at less than 3 kilometres per hour.

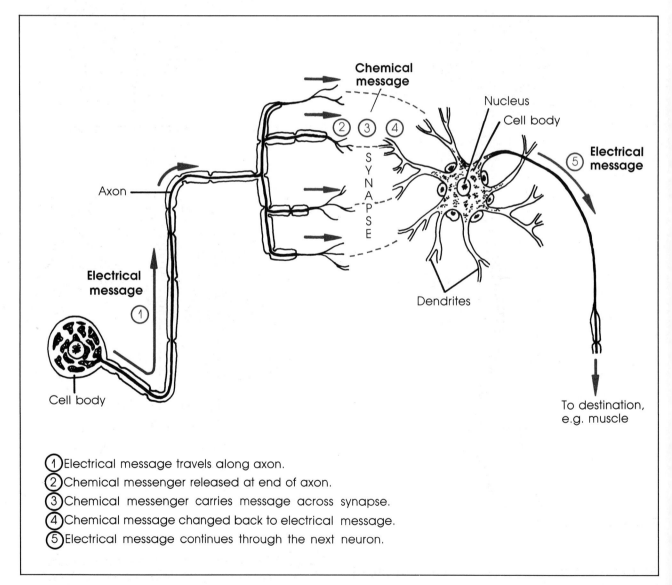

① Electrical message travels along axon.
② Chemical messenger released at end of axon.
③ Chemical messenger carries message across synapse.
④ Chemical message changed back to electrical message.
⑤ Electrical message continues through the next neuron.

**Figure 2.36:** The transmission of a message through the synapse.

# Divisions of the nervous system

The nervous system has two parts:
- The central nervous system – the brain and the spinal cord.
- The peripheral nervous system – all the nerves and nerve centres of the other parts of the body.

Nerves which carry messages from muscles and other body parts to the central nervous system are called *sensory* or *afferent* nerves; nerves which carry messages away from the central nervous system to muscles and other body parts are called *motor* or *efferent* nerves.

## The central nervous system

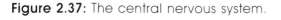

**Figure 2.37:** The central nervous system.

*The brain*

As the brain is so vital to the functioning of the body, it is securely protected. It is

located inside the skull and is covered by a membrane of very fine tissue. Under this membrane is a fluid which acts as a shock absorber to minimise damage if the skull is jolted. The brain weighs about 1.4 kilograms and looks like a grey, wrinkly, very soft mass.

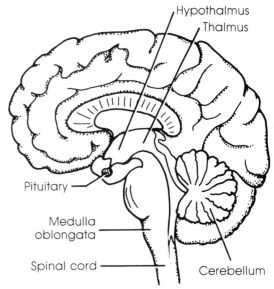

**Figure 2.38(a):** Cross-section of the brain.

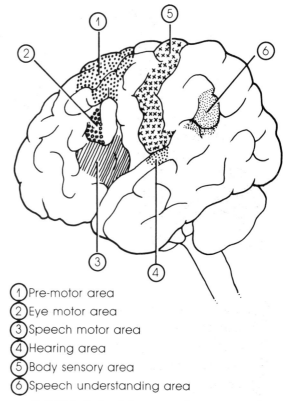

(1) Pre-motor area
(2) Eye motor area
(3) Speech motor area
(4) Hearing area
(5) Body sensory area
(6) Speech understanding area

**Figure 2.38(b):** Scientists are not sure exactly how the brain functions. This diagram shows areas whose functions they are fairly sure of.

The brain has three main divisions:

- The *cerebrum* is the largest part of the brain. Different parts of the cerebrum control:
  - voluntary movement of muscles
  - hearing, speaking and writing
  - awareness of pain, touch, temperature and smell
  - the ability to work out distance, size and shape.

  The cerebrum is the site of intelligence, thought, memory, artistic effort and emotions.
- The *medulla oblongata*, the area where the spinal cord joins the brain, controls automatic funtions such as breathing, heartbeat and digestion. Near the medulla is a network of neurons which control sleeping and waking.
- The *cerebellum* assists in controlling body movement. The cerebellum is able to store information about movement and can therefore make movement more precise, smoother, better balanced and better coordinated.

*The spinal cord*

The spinal cord is enclosed by the vertebral column. It runs from the lower brain to the pelvic area. It has two jobs: it can transmit messages to and from the brain and it can also be involved in reflex action.

## The autonomic nervous system

The autonomic nervous system is a specialised part of the nervous system. It controls involuntary body functions such as heartbeat, movement of smooth muscles (e.g. digestion), and the production of saliva and sweat.

### The peripheral nervous system

The peripheral nerves are all the nerves of the body not found in the central nervous system. There are two main groups of peripheral nerves:

- the cranial nerves
- the spinal nerves.

The twelve pairs of cranial nerves bring directly to the brain messages about pain, touch, temperature, pressure, smell, vision and hearing. They also carry out messages to move voluntary and involuntary muscles, to make organs such as the heart and lungs work and to activate glands.

The thirty-one pairs of spinal nerves branching out from the spinal cord carry messages to and from many areas of the body including skeletal muscles.

## Reflexes

Reflexes are involuntary responses to stimuli. The "knee jerk" is an example of a reflex action. If a person is tapped below the kneecap, a message is sent to the spinal cord which then transmits the message to a muscle in the thigh which contracts and jerks the lower leg upwards. Not all reflexes go through the spinal cord. If a light is shone into the eye, the pupil contracts in a reflex action.

# The endocrine system

The endocrine system is the chemical messenger system. We do not yet fully understand how it works.

## The functions of the endocrine system

With the nervous system, the endocrine system acts as a control and communications system. Whereas the nervous system deals with rapid control timed in seconds, the endocrine system controls long-term body changes which can take minutes, hours or even years. Examples of these body changes are growth and the control of blood-sugar levels. The endocrine system can also affect a person's emotions.

# The structure and workings of the endocrine system

The endocrine system consists of glands which secrete hormones (chemical messengers) and pass them into the blood stream which circulates them throughout the body.

## The pituitary gland

This pea-sized gland is found at the base of the brain. Although it secretes a growth hor-mone which regulates body growth during childhood, it is often referred to as the "master gland" because it also secretes hor-mones which control other glands.

## The thyroid gland

The thyroid gland is found in the neck. It secretes a hormone which controls body energy and assists in growth. It also helps control temperature.

## The parathyroids

These four glands are found behind the thyroid gland. The hormone from the parathyroids regulates the body's supply of calcium to ensure the proper functioning of digestion, and of heart, muscle and nerve action.

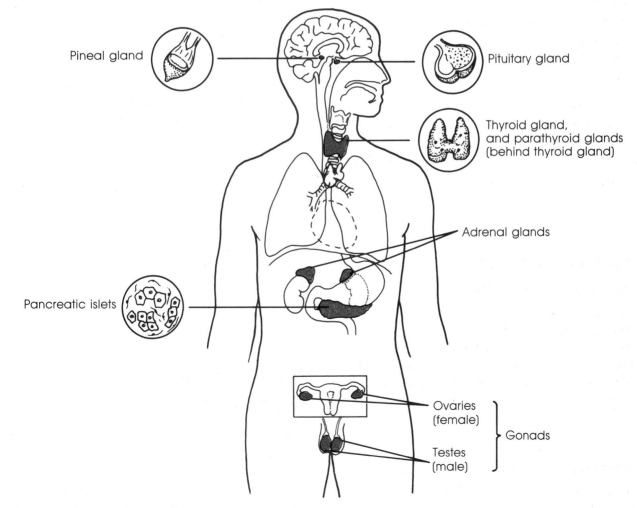

**Figure 2.39:** The glands of the endocrine system.

## The adrenal glands

The adrenal glands secrete several hormones:
- Adrenalin allows the body to "super-charge" in preparation for emergency action such as fighting or flight.
- Other secretions help control the amount of mineral salts in the body and the production of energy.

Apart from these glands, there are the gonads which regulate sexual development, the pineal gland which affects sexual development but whose function is not yet completely understood, and the pancreatic islets of the pancreas which secrete insulin to control the blood-sugar level.

# The skin system

The skin system consists of the skin, hair and nails.

## The functions of the skin system

The skin system:
- provides a waterproof covering protecting the body
- helps regulate body temperature
- excretes fluid
- manufactures vitamin D
- produces hair and an oil called sebum.

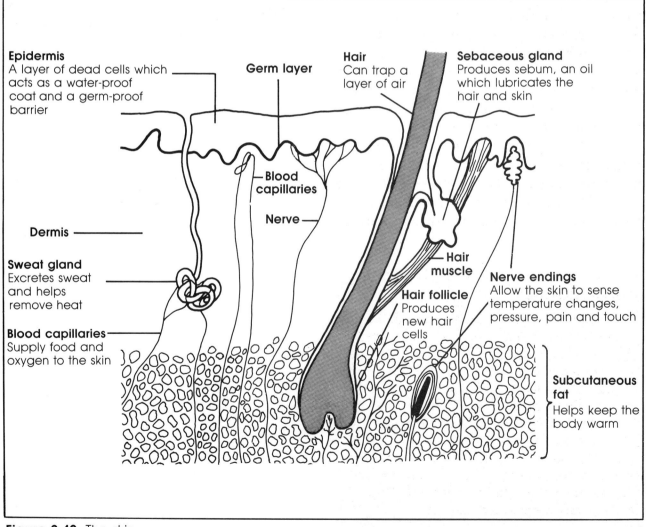

**Figure 2.40:** The skin.

# The structure and workings of the skin system

The organ of the skin system is the skin itself. Totally covering the body, it is the largest organ of the human body. The skin provides a tough cover preventing the passage of bacteria, water, fungi and most chemicals into the body.

Through sweat glands, the skin excretes perspiration. Although 99 per cent of perspiration is water, the other 1 per cent contains solid body waste which is mostly salt, some body acid and even some vitamins B and C.

Perspiration actually helps spread an antiseptic film over the skin. The skin helps maintain temperature as close to the body's normal 37°C as possible. In hot weather, the skin produces perspiration which evaporates, removing heat and cooling the body. In cold weather, the small blood vessels of the skin constrict and decrease circulation, and the warm blood is diverted to muscles and important organs to keep them warm.

The skin, when exposed to sunlight, manufactures vitamin D for bone growth and development. The skin provides the sense of touch, and receives and sends information on pressure, temperature and pain.

# Hair and nails

Hair is found on every part of the body except the palms of the hand and the soles of the feet. Hair consists of a root, located inside a follicle in the skin, and a long shaft. Inside the root, hair cells die and are pushed out from the root, making it appear as though the hair is growing. Although the hair itself is dead, it is kept in good condition by the oil glands in the follicle. Hair helps protect the body. It prevents dust and foreign bodies entering the nose and sometimes the ears. Eyebrows stop sweat dripping into the eyes. Hair also increases the body's sensitivity to touch.

Fingernails and toenails grow about 1 millimetre per week. If damaged or removed, they can regenerate; a fingernail takes about five months and a toenail about eight months to grow.

## Skin colour

Melanin is the pigment produced in the skin. It can colour the skin brown, black or yellow depending on racial origin. Sunlight increases the production of melanin, resulting in suntan. The colour of the skin is also affected by skin thickness and blood supply. Doctors are aided in diagnosis of disease by checking skin colour and skin conditions. Abnormally pale skin may be the result of anaemia; liver malfunction causes yellowish colour and rashes often show the presence of diseases such as chickenpox and measles.

# 3

# The body in movement

In order to improve your performance in sport, it is important for you to know:
- how movement occurs
- how to make a particular movement
- how to control that movement
- what factors can affect that movement.

The human body has often been described as a machine for doing work. To make sure that the "body machine" works most efficiently, it is helful to understand not only the operation of the body but also the laws of physics during activity.

Today, many athletes take videos of themselves to see how they perform, and then apply the principles of physics to improve their movement. Computers also have helped, in that they can provide diagrams to show the most efficient way of performing a skill. However, you must remember that individual athletes can still produce outstanding performances even when they use methods which are less efficient according to the laws of physics. The best way to improve your own performance is to be as fit as possible and to practise your skills to find the methods that suit you best.

# Movement

## Systems working together

When you move, many body systems are involved:
- Bones form the framework and provide the basis of a lever system.
- Joints enable the framework to bend.
- Muscles pull on bones to cause movement.
- The nervous system transmits messages to the muscles so that they can act.
- The circulatory system brings nutrients to the muscles, so that the muscles have the energy to work.
- The respiratory system provides oxygen.
- Other systems can also be involved: for example, the endocrine system can assist by secreting adrenalin; the skin system can increase the perspiration rate.

# The action of muscles

Muscles can be used for many types of movement. Movement occurs when a muscle contracts to pull on a bone and another muscle relaxes to allow that bone to move. For example, when you bend your elbow, your biceps are the prime movers which contract to pull on the bone, and your triceps are the antagonists which relax to allow movement to take place. When you straighten your arm again, the triceps contract and the biceps relax.

# Joints

Muscles could not cause movement if the joints did not allow the skeletal framework to bend. The freely moveable joints are the most important in movement. Table 3.1 shows the joints and their movements.

**Table 3.1:** Freely moveable joints and their movements

| Joint | Example | Movement |
|---|---|---|
| Ball and socket | Shoulder; hip | Wide range of movement |
| Hinge | Elbow; knee; finger | Movement in one direction only |
| Pivot | Head on to spine; elbow | Turning or rotating |
| Gliding | Carpal bones in wrist; tarsal bones in ankle | Limited movement |

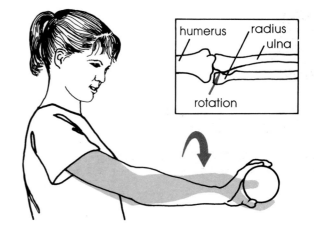

**Figure 3.1(c):** Pivot joint.

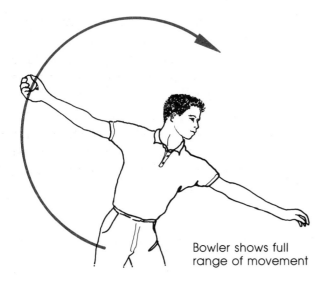

Bowler shows full range of movement

**Figure 3.1(a):** Ball and socket joint.

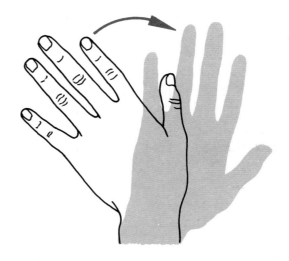

**Figure 3.1(d):** Gliding joint.

# Naming movement

## The anatomical position

To be able to name types of movement, you must have a reference position of the body. The reference position is called the anatomical position. It exists when a person stands without moving, head to the front, feet shoulder-width apart and arms held slightly away from the sides with palms facing forwards. All movement can be described from this position.

When a person moves from the anatomical position, muscles, bones and joints work together to allow twisting, turning, bending,

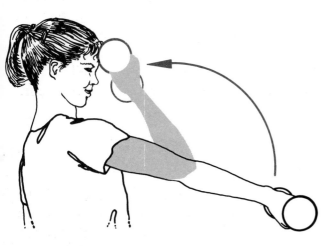

**Figure 3.1(b):** Hinge joint.

straightening and rotating. These movements are given special names.

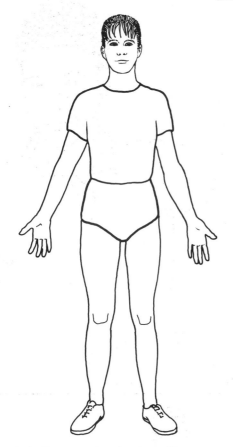

**Figure 3.2:** The anatomical position.

## Types of movement

There are six main types of movement that are caused by muscle action.

**Flexion** is a movement which *bends*, thereby decreasing the angle at the joint between bones. The prime movers in flexion are the flexors (see figure 3.3).

**Extension** is a movement which *straightens*, thereby increasing the angle at the joint between bones. It is the opposite of flexion. The prime movers in extension are extensors (figure 3.4).

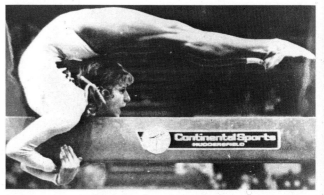

Hyperextension occurs when a joint is extended beyond its normal limit. This gymnast must take great care not to harm the joints in the back bone.

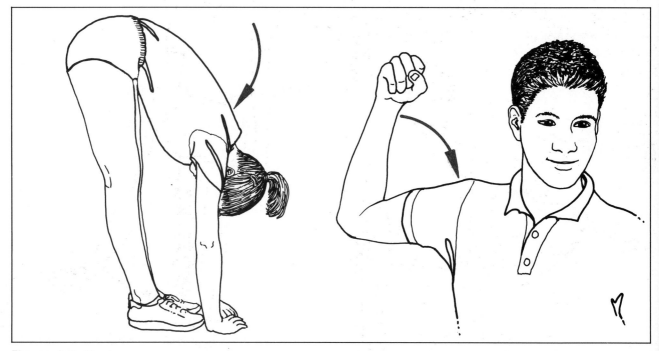

**Figure 3.3:** Flexion.

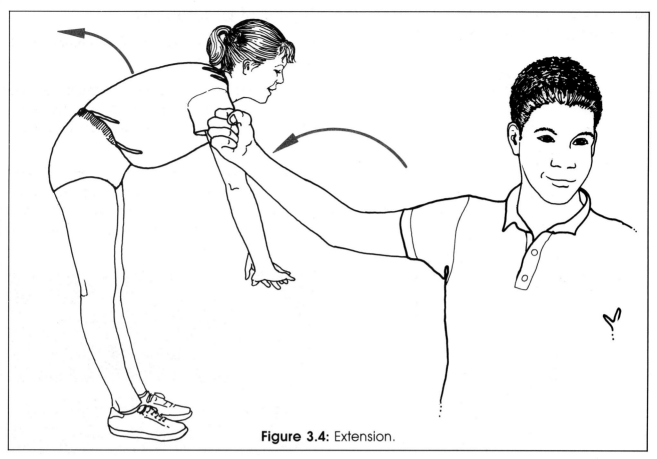

**Figure 3.4:** Extension.

**Abduction** is a movement of a bone *away from* the centre line of the body. The prime movers in abduction are abductors.

**Adduction** is a movement *towards* the centre line of the body. It is the opposite of abduction. The prime movers in adduction are adductors.

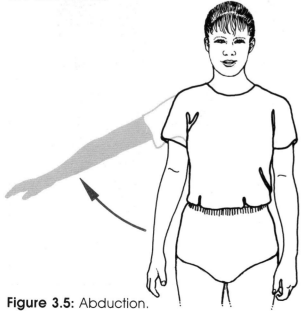

**Figure 3.5:** Abduction.

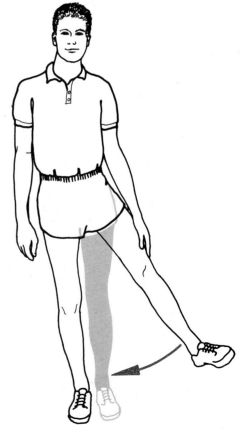

**Figure 3.6:** Adduction.

**Rotation** is a movement where the bone is moved *around* a central axis.

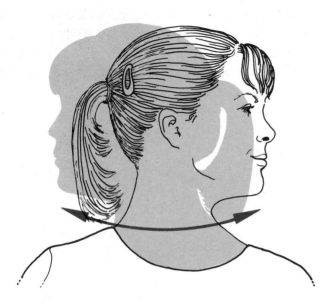

**Figure 3.7:** Rotation.

**Circumduction** is a movement where the end of the bone makes a *circle*. A cone shape is formed.

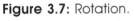

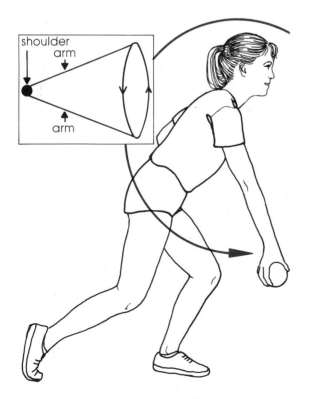

**Figure 3.8:** Circumduction.

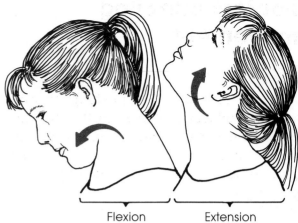

Flexion          Extension

Rotation

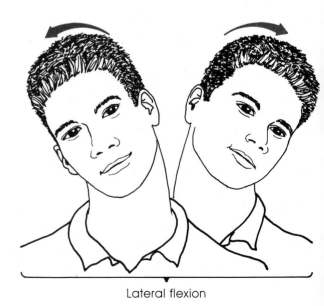

Lateral flexion

**Figure 3.9:** Movements of the head and neck.

# Factors affecting movement

## Force

Force is the action of pushing or pulling which produces a change in the movement of an object. Force can be applied to a body at rest or to one in motion. There are two types of force which influence your physical performance:

- Internal forces come from within the human body. They are caused by actions of muscles, ligaments, bones and other body tissue.
- External forces come from outside the body. Examples are gravity, friction, resistance and forces exerted by other bodies.

Force is measured in newtons.

## Forces at work

### Levers and the body

Levers are simple machines. "[They] are rigid bars which can rotate or turn about a fixed point when force or effort is applied to overcome some resistance."*

Levers must have:

- an effort point ($E$) – the place where force is applied.
- a pivot point ($P$) – the place about which the rigid bar can turn. (This is also called a fulcrum.)
- a resistance point ($R$) – the place where the force being applied is resisted.

Levers can be used:

- to maintain balance
- to use less effort to overcome heavy lifting
- to give a wider range of movement
- to give greater speed to an object.

One way of regarding the human body is to see it as consisting of levers which can perform work. Your arms, legs, fingers, toes, jaw, neck, back and hips can all be used as levers.

---

*Wells and Luttgens, *Kinesiology* (Philadelphia: Saunders, 1976)

Levers come in three types – Class I, Class II and Class III levers.

*Class I levers*

In Class I levers, the pivot point lies between the effort point and the resistance point. Depending on the position of the pivot, the resistance point will be given either greater speed or greater force.

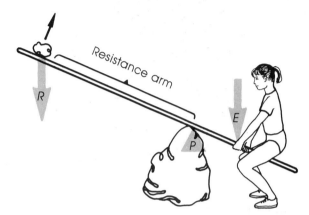

**Figure 3.10(a):** In this situation, the longer resistance arm of the lever allows for increased speed.

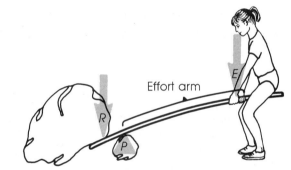

**Figure 3.10(b):** In this situation, the longer effort arm allows for increased force which means the heavy object can be moved more easily.

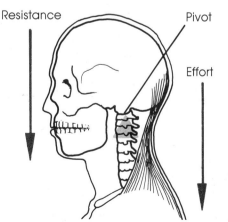

**Figure 3.11:** A Class I lever keeps the head upright and balanced.

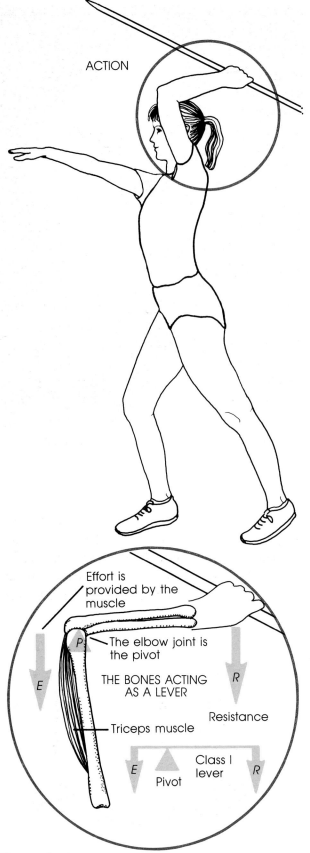

ACTION

Effort is provided by the muscle

P — The elbow joint is the pivot

THE BONES ACTING AS A LEVER

E

R

Resistance

Triceps muscle

E   Class I lever   R

Pivot

**Figure 3.12:** In throwing the javelin, a Class I lever is formed by the forearm and the elbow joint. This lever increases speed.

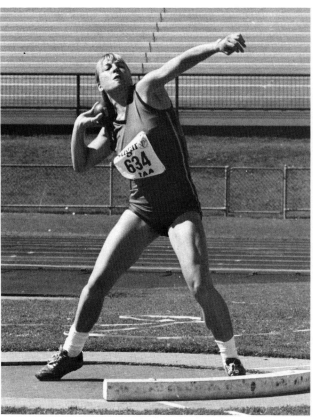

A Class I lever in action.

## Class II levers

In Class II levers, the pivot point is at one end, the effort point is at the other end, and the resistance point lies between. Class II levers favour force rather than speed because the effort arm is longer than the resistance arm.

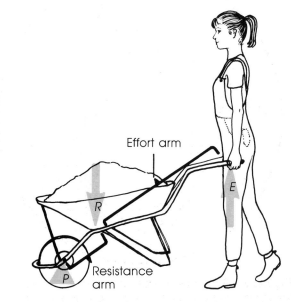

Effort arm

R

E

P   Resistance arm

**Figure 3.13:** A Class II lever used to lift a load.

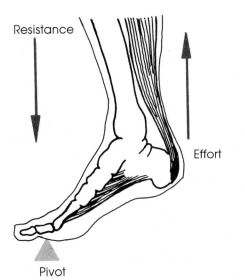

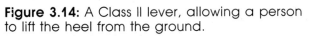

**Figure 3.14:** A Class II lever, allowing a person to lift the heel from the ground.

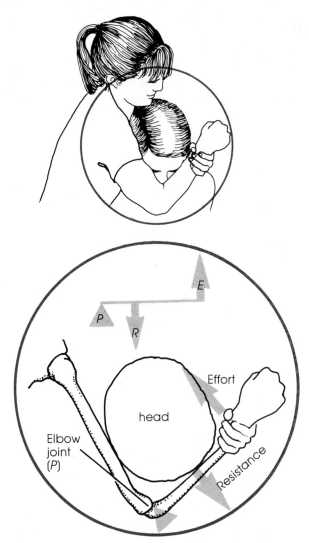

**Figure 3.15:** In this wrestling headlock, the forearm and elbow form a Class II lever to create increased force.

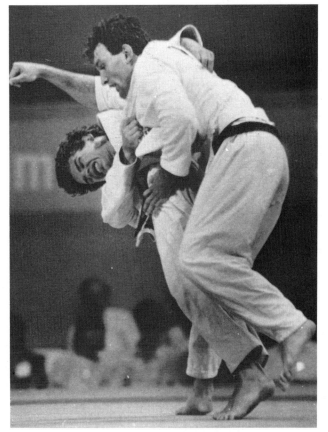

In judo, Class II levers are frequently used.

### Class III levers

In Class III levers, the pivot point is at one end, the resistance point is at the other end, and the effort point is in between. Class III levers favour speed rather than force because the resistance arm is longer than the effort arm.

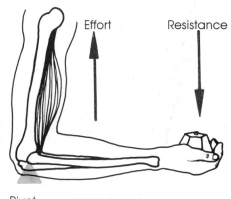

**Figure 3.16:** This Class III lever allows a person to hold an object steadily.

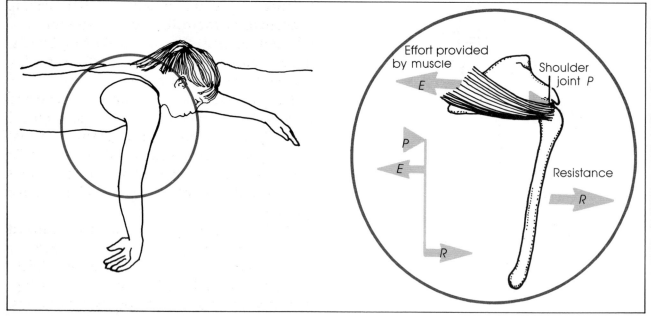

**Figure 3.17:** In swimming, a Class III lever is formed by the shoulder joint and the bone of the upper arm to increase speed.

Most body levers are Class III levers that are used to increase speed or distance rather than force. They have the effort (muscle) between the pivot (joint) and the resistance (extremity).

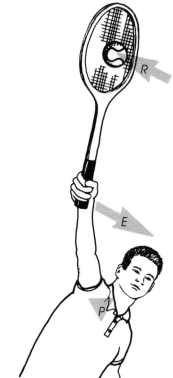

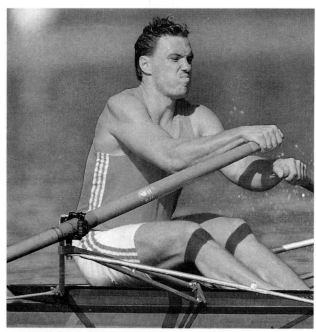

A Class III lever in action.

The body's levers can be made even more effective by using bats, racquets, oars and other equipment to increase the length of the natural lever.

**Figure 3.18:** Most striking implements such as bats, racquets and clubs form Class III levers. The implements become extensions of the body's bone levers. Here the tennis racquet is an extension of the full arm and together they act as one lever. The shoulder joint is the pivot; the muscles of the arm and body provide effort. If the whole lever, racquet and arm, is swung faster, the ball can be hit harder. But performance is lessened if the elbow is bent causing the length of the lever to decrease.

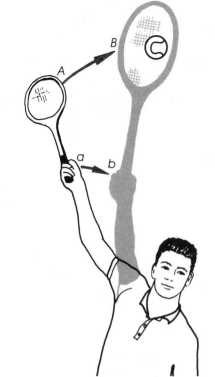

**Figure 3.19:** The time taken for the hand to move from a to b is the same as that for the racquet to move from A to B. Therefore, the speed of the racquet is much faster than the speed of the hand. This principle can be applied in cricket, hockey, baseball and golf.

## Gravity

Gravity is the force by which the earth pulls all objects towards it. Gravity gives your body and other objects weight. It stops you, or a ball kicked by you, from floating off into space. Gravity is particularly important in sport because:

- it is an external force which many athletes have combat by developing internal forces. The high jumper, the runner, the footballer, the gymnast and the basketballer all have to fight gravity with muscle power to perform well.
- it is a force which aids some sports. Gravity is essential to such sports as high diving, sky diving, downhill skiing and tobogganing.
- it affects balance.

## Balance

One of the most important factors influencing your performance in sport is good balance. If you are off-balance when playing basketball or football, you will stumble and fall. For the sprinter in the starting blocks, the gymnast or the springboard diver, having correct balance is essential.

Being balanced depends on your centre of gravity. Your centre of gravity when you are standing in the anatomical position is just above your navel. In males it is usually 56 per cent of height above ground; in females it is usually 54 per cent of height above ground.

The line of gravity is an imaginary vertical line drawn through the body's centre of gravity to the base of support (figure 3.20(a)). In the anatomical position, your base of support is your two feet. If you lean sideways, backwards or forwards, your centre of gravity will shift (figure 3.20(b), p. 52). If you lean over far enough, your centre of gravity will shift outside your base of support and you will fall over (figure 3.20(c)).

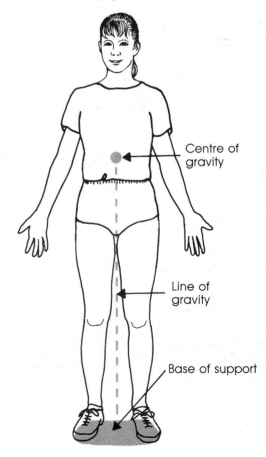

Centre of gravity

Line of gravity

Base of support

**Figure 3.20(a):** The line of gravity in the anatomical position.

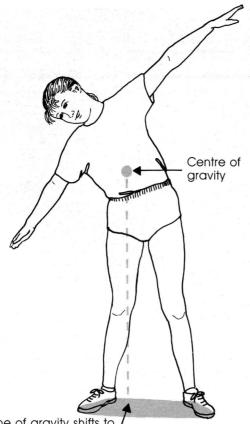

Centre of gravity

Line of gravity shifts to edge of base of support

**Figure 3.20(b):** The line of gravity shifts to the edge of the base of support when you lean a little.

*Ways to maintain balance*

There are three factors to remember when performing a sport which requires good balance:

- To remain balanced, you must keep your line of gravity within the base of support.
- The larger your base of support, the more stable your body. You can increase your base of support merely by putting your feet further apart or by using your hands.

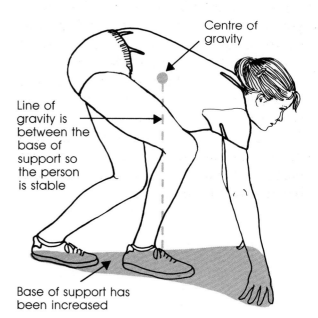

Centre of gravity

Line of gravity is between the base of support so the person is stable

Base of support has been increased

**Figure 3.21:** A sprinter is more stable in this starting position than standing upright and leaning over.

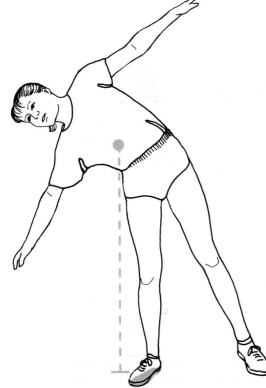

**Figure 3.20(c):** The line of gravity moves outside the base of support if you lean too far.

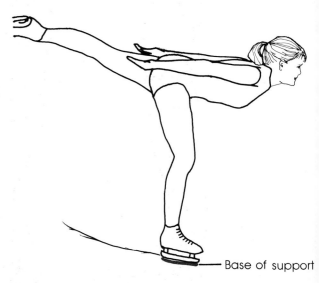

Base of support

**Figure 3.22:** Maintaining balance with outstretched arms and leg when the base of support is small.

In some sports such as figure-skating and gymnastics you are often required to keep your base of support very small to increase the difficulty of the movement and thus gain higher points. A skater uses an outstretched leg and arms to maintain balance.

- The lower your centre of gravity, the more stable your body. If you shift your centre of gravity upwards by raising your arms, you may become unbalanced. If you bend your knees, you bring your centre of gravity closer to your base of support and your balance will improve.

This is an important factor to remember in sports such as basketball and football where a knock can throw you off-balance. It is also important in sports such as gymnastics and skiing. If you begin to lose balance, crouch down a little and your balance will be improved.

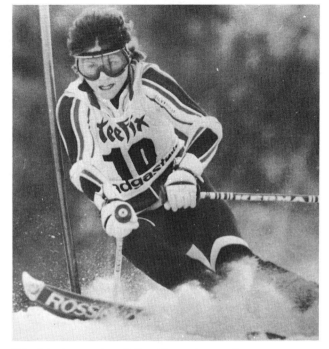

World champion Erika Hess shows the importance of correct balance as she speeds to victory on the slalom course.

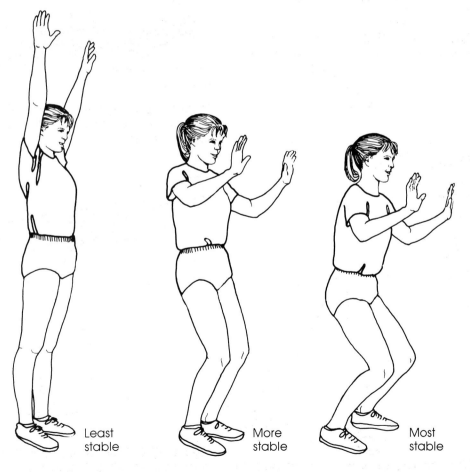

Least stable    More stable    Most stable

**Figure 3.23:** The lower the centre of gravity, the more stable your body.

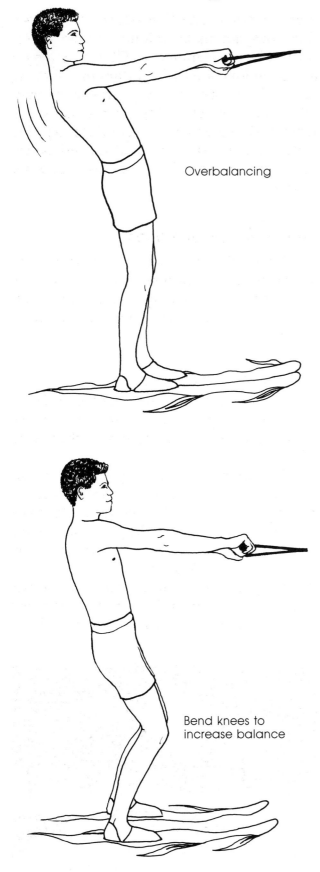

Overbalancing

Bend knees to
increase balance

**Figure 3.24:** In skiing, bent knees will help to
maintain your balance.

## Motion

Motion involves a change of position of an
object. Changes in motion occur when force
is applied. In sport, there are two types of
motion:

● *Linear motion.* This occurs when a person
or an object moves in a straight line. For
example, runners, swimmers, skiers and
divers move in linear motion; so do tennis
and golf balls.

● *Rotary motion.* This occurs when a person
or an object moves about a fixed point
called the pivot. Examples of rotary
motion are a gymnast performing a giant
swing on the high bar, a person doing sit-
ups, or the discus thrower turning before
releasing the discus.

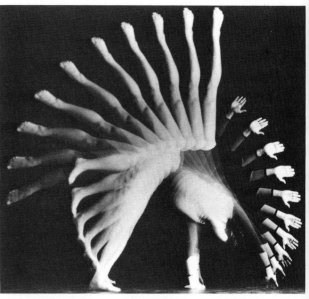

The rapid cycle of movements during
gymnastics is captured here using a special
flash unit. The result shows a perfect example
of rotary movement of the gymnast's body in a
cartwheel.

Most movement in sport is a combination
of both linear and rotary motion. The discus
thrower moves in rotary motion, but the
discus itself moves in both linear and rotary
motion; the footballer uses rotary motion to
kick the ball and the ball moves in linear
motion and often in rotary motion as well.

## Factors affecting motion

You will find many things affect your ability to move in the direction in which you want to go and at the speed at which you want to travel. Gravity, air and water resistance are the most important factors affecting motion in sport.

**Air resistance.** In physical activity, there are two types of air resistance important to you:

- the natural air resistance which works against all moving objects. This resistance causes a "drag", which helps slow down objects in the air. The larger and more upright the object, the greater the resistance. Thus cyclists lean low over the cycle to streamline themselves to minimise drag. However, air resistance can also aid objects in flight by providing "lift".
- the wind factor. When it is windy, athletes must take the force of the wind into account. For example, a person running into the wind is slowed; a runner is helped by a tail wind. In team sports, such as football or hockey, the captain who wins the toss often chooses to run into the wind in the early part of the game when players are fresh and to have the wind behind the team in the later stages of the game when the players are tired. However, sometimes captains choose to use the wind factor early in case the wind drops.

**Water resistance** also causes friction on an object or person passing through it. Water resistance is stronger than air resistance; this is one reason that runners can go faster than swimmers.

The effect of water resistance can be decreased if a person is more buoyant. Buoyancy is the ability to float. A swimmer with high buoyancy is able to swim more on the surface of the water than one who has low buoyancy. Women are slightly more buoyant than men, and plump people are more buoyant than thin people. Of course, this does not make thinner people necessarily slower swimmers. Fitness, strength and technique are all important in achieving speed. You should also remember that, when you are swimming, you actually use water resistance to pull yourself through the water. If the water provided no resistance, you would merely flap your arms and get nowhere.

## Newton's laws of motion

Sir Isaac Newton was a scientist who described motion in three laws. These laws can be applied to all motion in sport and can be used to make your techniques more efficient.

### *The first law of motion*

"A body remains in a state of rest (inertia) or uniform motion in a straight line unless acted upon by external forces to change its state."

This laws means that any change in the motion of an object is caused by a force.

- A golf ball must be hit into the air to make it move. It slows and drops to the ground because the forces of gravity and air resistance work on it.
- High jumpers use internal force to propel themselves upwards. Gravity and air resistance return them to the ground.

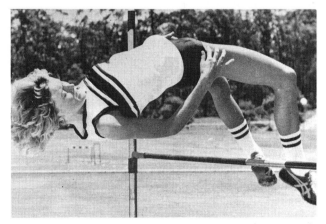

Internal force is needed to fight against the force of gravity.

- Runners waiting in a crouch start are preparing to use internal force to propel themselves forward.

*The second law of motion*

"The acceleration of a body is proportional to the force acting upon it."

This law provides us with two important relationships in sport:

- Force is equal to mass by acceleration $(F = ma)$.
  - The greater the mass, the more force is needed to provide the same acceleration. You need more muscle power to put a shot as fast as you can throw a tennis ball.
  - In tennis, the greater the muscular force applied to hitting the ball, the greater the acceleration of the ball.
- Every moving body has momentum. It is measured by multiplying the mass of the moving body by its velocity $(M = mV)$. Thus the momentum of a moving object depends on its mass and speed. The heavier a moving object, the greater its momentum; the faster a body moves, the greater its momentum. In order to change momentum, a force has to be applied to the moving body.
  - If you weigh 50 kg and are running at 10 m/s, then your momentum is 500 kg m/s.
  - A light object will have to move with greater speed than a heavy object if the momentum is to be the same.
  - A heavy footballer running at the same speed as a lighter footballer can knock him over in a collision. However, a lighter footballer running very fast can knock over a heavy, slower player because the faster runner develops more momentum. Players in contact sports should be aware of the part momentum can play in causing injury; it is possible for a faster, lighter player to cause more damage than a heavy, slow player.

# Choosing a bat applying Newton's laws

A batter often wants to hit a ball as fast and therefore as far as possible. The weight of the bat affects this. Look at table 3.2. In this example, the player used bats of different weights and swung the bat at the same speed each time. As you can see, the heavier the bat, the faster the ball travelled when hit.

**Table 3.2:** Different weights of bat, same speed

| Weight of bat | Speed of ball after hit (in metres/sec) |
|---|---|
| 0.57 kg | 30.6 |
| 0.71 kg | 32.6 |
| 0.85 kg | 34.0 |
| 0.99 kg | 35.1 |
| 1.14 kg | 35.9 |

However, the weight of the bat is only one factor involved in hitting a ball as fast and as far as possible. Look at table 3.3. In this example, the batter used a 0.85 kg bat and varied the speed of the swing. The speed with which the bat was swung made a difference. The faster the speed of swing, the faster the speed of the ball after it is hit.

**Table 3.3:** Same weight of bat, different speeds

| Speed bat was swung (in metres/sec) | Speed of ball after hit (in metres/sec) |
|---|---|
| 9.2 | 27.7 |
| 12.2 | 30.7 |
| 15.3 | 34.0 |
| 18.3 | 37.4 |
| 21.4 | 40.8 |

Now compare the two tables. The batter was able to hit the ball faster with the 0.85 kg bat than with the heavier 1.14 kg bat because the speed of swing was faster.

Thus, choosing a bat with a weight that is right for you is very important in achieving a better performance. If you choose a bat that is too heavy, your swing will be slowed and therefore so will the speed of the ball. However, through training and strengthening of muscles, you may be able to swing a heavier bat at the same speed as a lighter bat and therefore increase ball speed.

*The third law of motion*

"For every action there is an equal and opposite reaction."

- When a sprinter pushes against the starting blocks, the blocks in turn exert the same force back to the sprinter.

- For a swimmer to move forward more quickly through the water, the arms must push the water backwards. If, in freestyle, you use too much force on the downward part of your stroke as the arm enters the water, the rest of your body will move upwards; and if you use too much force at the end of the stroke as the arm leaves the water, the rest of the body will move down. These two actions will create an up-and-down bobbing effect, which will cause you to swim more slowly and waste a lot of effort.

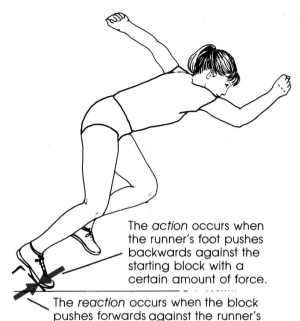

The *action* occurs when the runner's foot pushes backwards against the starting block with a certain amount of force.

The *reaction* occurs when the block pushes forwards against the runner's foot with the same amount of force.

**Figure 3.25:** Newton's third law — action and reaction.

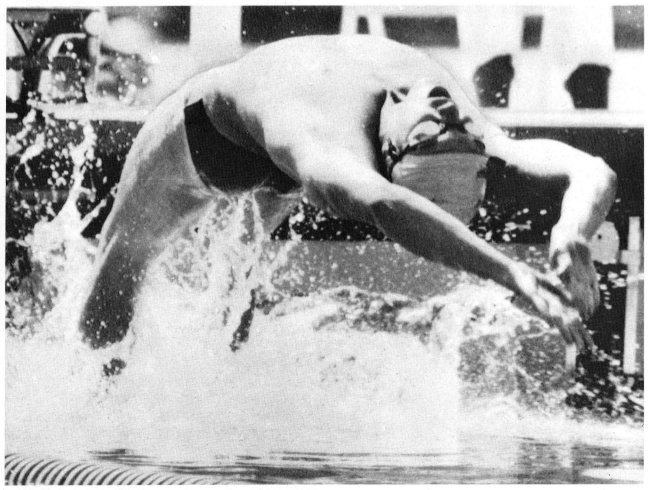

The backstroke start shows Newton's third law in action. The more force you apply to the wall the further you can thrust away from the wall.

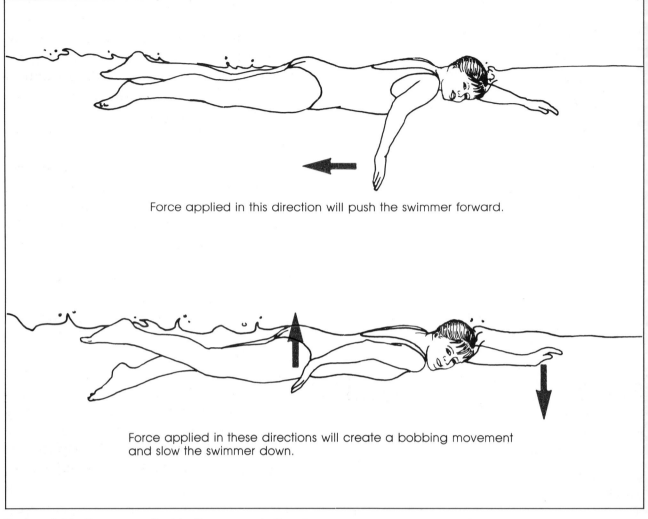

Force applied in this direction will push the swimmer forward.

Force applied in these directions will create a bobbing movement and slow the swimmer down.

**Figure 3.26:** Force applied in the correct direction will help you to swim faster.

# The use of momentum and motion

In sports, we are constantly trying to improve the distance, the speed or the accuracy of an object or ourselves. The distance we can hit or throw an object depends on:

- the speed at which the object is released. The faster the ball is thrown or hit, the further it will go.
- the angle at which the object is released. If the angle is too high, the object may go high but not far. If the angle is too low, the object will hit the ground too early. Under normal conditions, 45° is approximately the best angle at which to release the object to attain maximum distance.
- the distance over which the force is applied. Thus, javelin throwers and fast bowlers use long approaches to increase the speed of the javelin or cricket ball when it leaves their hands.
- the time during which the force acts. The longer a golf club is in contact with a ball, the faster the ball will travel after it has been hit. A small force applied to an object over a longer time can make that object go as fast as can a larger force applied to it for a shorter time.

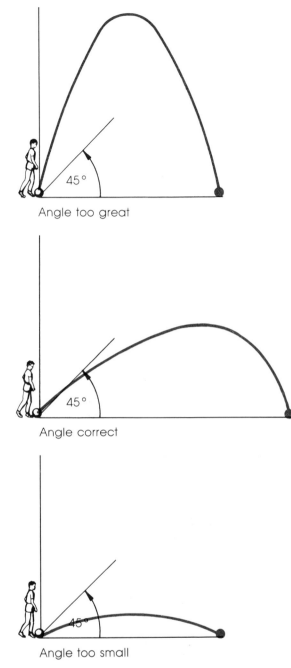

Angle too great

Angle correct

Angle too small

**Figure 3.27:** The angle at which at object is released affects the distance attained.

## Stopping an object

Deceleration or slowing down of an object or yourself is very important in sport. Many people have been hurt because they have not known how to stop a ball correctly or how to stop themselves. There are two important aspects to deceleration: force and pressure.

To catch a ball most effectively, the force of the ball must be absorbed, otherwise it will bounce out of your hand. One way to absorb the force of a ball is to increase the time or distance it travels once it reaches your hand. For example, if you bend your elbow as you catch a cricket ball, the impact is lessened and you are more likely to hang on to the ball. In some sports, gloves filled with sponge rubber help to absorb the force of the ball.

When a ball is caught in your hand, you feel a certain amount of pressure. Pressure is the force of the ball over a certain area. The smaller the area of contact, the greater the pressure; the greater the area of contact, the smaller the pressure. Thus, a second way to absorb the force of the ball is to increase the area of contact with the ball. Using two hands instead of one doubles the area of absorption and allows you to hold on to the ball more easily.

The technique of decreasing force and pressure is also applied when an athlete wants to stop: the sprinter gradually slows down after the end of a race; the baseballer slides along the ground to the base; the parachutist bends the knees or rolls over when landing.

## Posture

Your posture is the way you hold your body upright whether you are sitting, standing or walking. Poor posture causes muscle and ligament strain and can even lead to problems such as stiff neck, headaches, back ache, and displacement of internal organs.

There is no single correct posture for everyone, but there are guidelines that you can follow. Good posture reduces tiredness, improves coordination and increases general health and confidence.

## Good posture when standing

Figure 3.28 on page 60 illustrates several standing postures, and the points listed

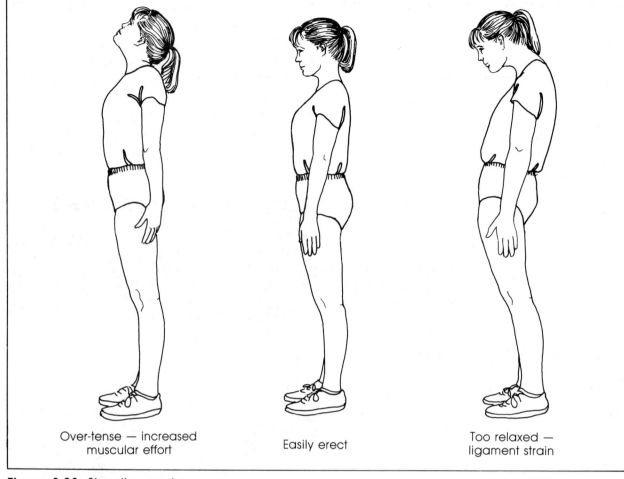

Over-tense — increased muscular effort

Easily erect

Too relaxed — ligament strain

**Figure 3.28:** Standing postures.

below indicate things to keep in mind for good posture.

- Feet comfortably apart, weight evenly balanced, toes facing ahead.
- Knees straight and relaxed, neither bent nor forced back.
- Pelvis level and balanced over feet.
- Abdomen flat.
- Chest slightly up and forward.
- Shoulders straight, held easily not stiffly.
- Head balanced over body; chin in, back and neck stretched upwards.

# Good posture when sitting

Figure 3.29 illustrates good posture when seated.

- Feet flat on floor, knees bent at approximately 90 degrees.
- Height of seat should be adjusted to correspond to length of lower legs.

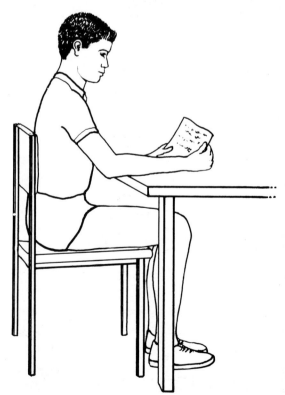

**Figure 3.29:** Posture when seated.

- Seat horizontal or with slight backward lean.
- The seat should support thighs close to back of knee but should not contact back of knee, as this may place unnecessary pressure on the major blood vessels.
- When writing at a desk it is necessary to bend forwards, but a back rest is important to occasionally support the trunk.
- Desk height should allow forearms to rest comfortably without effort from the shoulder muscles.
- There is no perfect sitting position. There are a number of good positions to choose from and a good chair should allow a person to adopt different positions to shift the load on joints and muscles.

## Good posture when walking

Figure 3.30 illustrates good posture when walking.

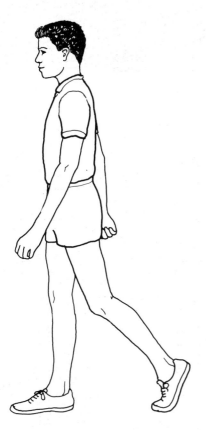

**Figure 3.30:** Good posture when walking.

- Toes pointed ahead, feet parallel or with slight out-toeing.
- Even, natural, rhythmic step.
- Swing arms easily and naturally.
- Carry head tall and straight, without straining.
- Avoid dragging legs or feet.
- Walk purposefully and with confidence.

## Importance of the feet

Feet allow us to walk and run. Yet feet are small in surface area. Any alteration in foot surface or awkward placing of the feet can affect body posture. Poorly fitting shoes worn over long periods can cause postural and feet problems.

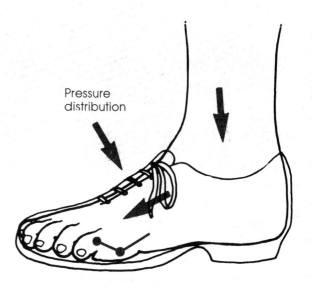

Pressure distribution

**Figure 3.31:** Calluses and corns are caused by pressure from poor foot mechanics or ill-fitting shoes. Poorly designed footwear can change normal foot function, and excessive wearing of badly fitting shoes, sandals or boots may lead to structural alterations in the foot.

Foot structure varies among people, although these variations do not usually cause problems. One variation is commonly called "flat feet". When most people put their foot on the ground, there is a space about a finger-width called an arch between the mid-foot and the floor. If fingers cannot be slipped into this space because the foot does not arch, the foot is called "flat" (see figure 3.32). "Flat feet" normally do not cause problems; however, if a person with "flat feet" suffers pain or fatigue during physical activity, a doctor should be consulted.

# Lifting posture

To prevent the possibility of injury when lifting:
- keep the back straight
- bend at the hips and knees, keeping the load close to the body. Do not bend *over* the load.

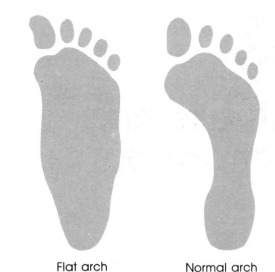

Flat arch        Normal arch

**Figure 3.32:** Arches of the feet.

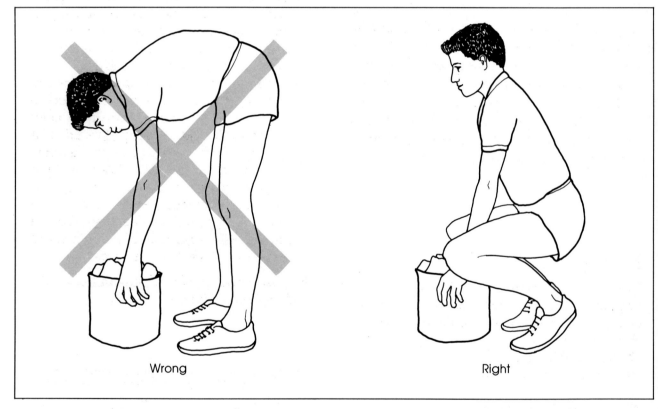

Wrong        Right

**Figure 3.33:** Lifting posture.

# Fitness and performance

Improving performance in sport depends on:
- developing proper training programmes
- physical fitness.

As physical fitness means different things to different people, it is probably better to talk about *levels* of fitness. The basic level of fitness is the ability to carry out everyday activities with ease and comfort; the top level of fitness is that reached by professional athletes or Olympians – a fitness which gives maximum body performance. This chapter is concerned with reaching a level of fitness that allows you to achieve your own peak performance in sport or recreation.

## Energy

Every physical activity requires energy. In physical fitness we must look at the sorts of energy available to muscles. Energy is available through:
- the aerobic system
- the anaerobic system.

### The aerobic system

The aerobic system is the most important energy system in everyday life. It is the system which provides energy for prolonged activity. It is called "aerobic" because it uses oxygen brought to the muscle cells from the heart–lung system. With this oxygen, the cells can process fuel to produce high levels of energy.

### The anaerobic system

The anaerobic system produces energy without the presence of oxygen in two ways:
- A substance called creatine phosphate (CP) is stored in the muscles. It can provide energy for efforts which involve short periods of activity of up to 10 seconds, such as lifting weights.
- A substance called glycogen is stored in the muscle cells. It is broken down to produce energy and a waste product called lactic acid. Although less efficient in producing energy than the aerobic system, glycogen breakdown without oxygen provides enough energy for short-term, intense effort such as a 200-metre sprint. It can also provide energy for acceleration of effort in sprint finishes of long-distance races.

In most sports, you draw on both the aerobic and anaerobic systems.

## The components of fitness

Although every sport has one particular part or component of fitness which is more important than another, to achieve all-round fitness the following components are essential:
- endurance
- strength
- flexibility
- power
- speed
- agility
- balance
- reaction time
- coordination.

# Endurance

Endurance is the most important component of fitness for an athlete. It means being able to continue physical activity for a long time. The fitter the athlete, the greater the level of endurance. Endurance comes from:

● cardio-vascular endurance
● muscular endurance.

## Cardio-vascular endurance

Cardio-vascular endurance is sometimes referred to as cardio-respiratory endurance because it involves the lungs, the heart, the blood and the blood vessels. It is the ability to exercise the whole body for long periods of time without running out of breath or becoming tired. An athlete with good cardio-vascular endurance usually has:

● a stronger heart
● a slower pulse rate which means the heart does not have to beat as often
● lower blood pressure
● larger lung capacity allowing more oxygen to be taken up by the blood.

An efficient cardio-vascular system increases aerobic and anaerobic endurance.

## Aerobic endurance

Aerobic endurance depends on the cardio-vascular system providing oxygen to the cells to produce energy. The more oxygen available to the muscles, the more energy can be produced and the less fatigue is felt. Thus, aerobic endurance depends on cardio-vascular endurance.

## Anaerobic endurance

Anaerobic endurance refers to the athlete's ability to draw on energy stored in the muscles, without the use of oxygen. When exercise is short and intense as in sprinting, the athlete has to rely on the immediate anaerobic energy available. For most people, this energy doesn't last long, approximately one minute. Trained athletes, however, are more efficient in drawing on anaerobic energy effectively.

## Muscular endurance

Muscular endurance is the ability to use the same muscles repeatedly without getting tired. For instance, in running long distances, the muscles of the legs are continuously being worked. Long-distance runners, swimmers, rowers and cyclists must have good muscular endurance.

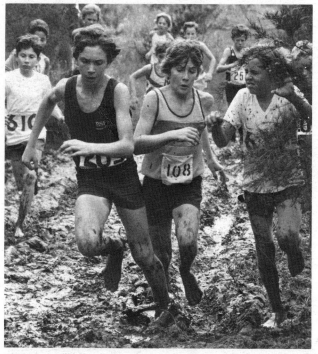

Cardio-vascular endurance is the basic component of fitness.

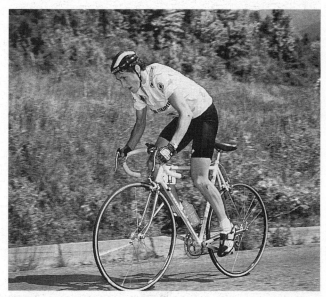

Muscular endurance is needed to cycle long distances.

# Strength

Strength refers to the amount of force exerted by muscles. This depends on:
- size of muscle
- ability of the nervous system to activate the muscle
- good coordination.

Strength is important in most sports.

# Flexibility

Flexibility is the ability to use muscles through their full range of movement and to move joints with ease. Being able to bend, stretch or twist easily indicates a high level of flexibility. This improves performance and lessens the risk of muscle injury and soreness. Flexibility is therefore important in all sports.

# Power

Power is the ability to release maximum force very quickly. It is a combination of speed and strength. Highjumpers, discus throwers and sprinters all need to have power.

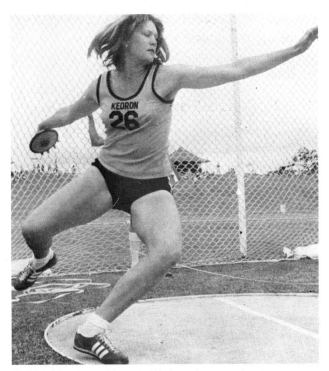

Discus throwers must have power.

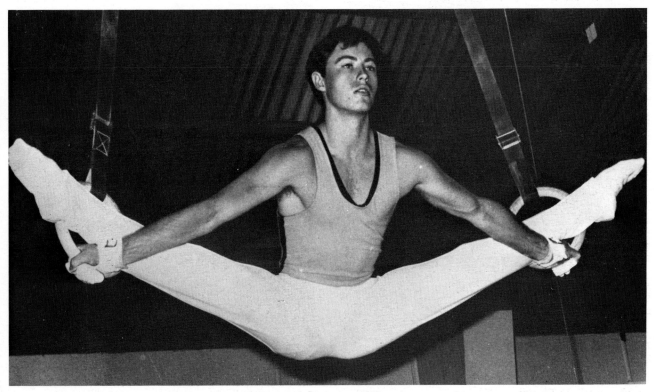

Gymnasts must have a high level of flexibility and strength.

# Speed

Speed is the ability to perform a movement or cover a distance in a short period of time. Speed can refer to total body speed, as in running or swimming, or rate of movement of body parts, such as leg speed or arm speed.

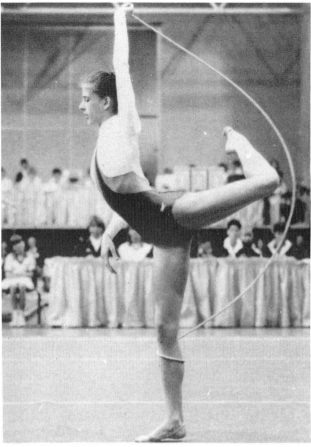

This gymnast shows a combination of flexibility, coordination and balance.

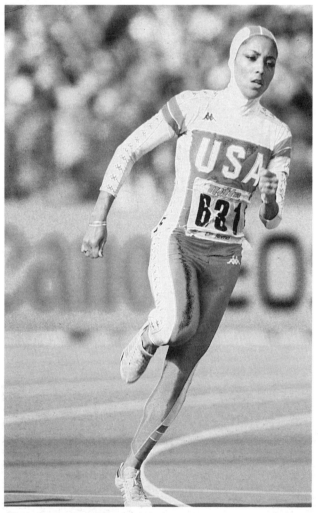

Sprinters need speed.

# Agility, balance, reaction time and coordination

**Agility** is the ability to move and change direction quickly. Wrestlers, footballers, gymnasts and fencers must all be agile.

**Balance** is the ability to remain stable even when moving. Gymnasts and surfers must have a high level of balance.

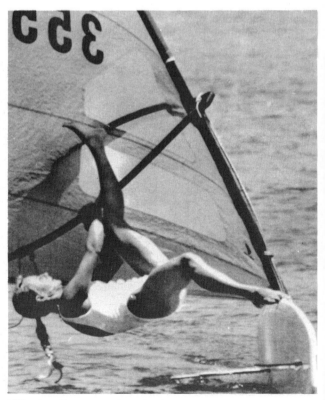

Windsurfing requires balance.

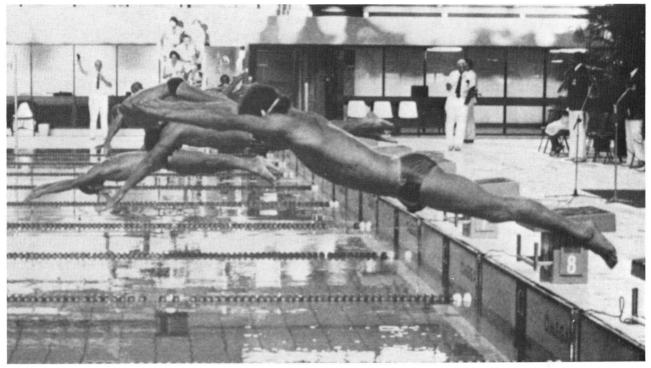

Note the different reaction times of these swimmers.

**Reaction time** is the amount of time it takes to make a physical response once you see the need to take an action. Good reaction time is needed in the starting blocks, in fencing and karate, and when defending a penalty in soccer or hockey.

**Coordination** is the linking of the senses such as sight and hearing through the brain to parts of the body to produce smooth, quick and efficiently controlled movement. Good coordination is necessary in all sports and is essential in bat and racquet sports.

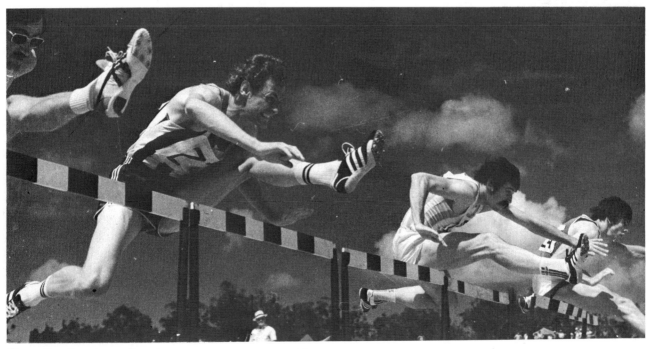

Coordination in action.

# Assessing and improving your fitness level

To improve your fitness, you should:
- assess your level of each component of fitness through standard tests
- increase or maintain that level by choosing exercises through the principles of specificity, overloading and reversibility.

## Specificity
Specificity means selecting exercises whose major purpose is to develop one component of fitness, such as cardio-vascular endurance or strength.

## Overloading
Overloading is extremely important in improving performance. Overloading means increasing the effort and work of your muscular and endurance systems until those systems are working hard. This can be achieved by gradually increasing:
- how hard you train (intensity)
- how long you train (duration)
- how often you train (frequency).

## Reversibility
Reversibility is a drop in level of fitness owing to lack of training. Regardless of how fit you may be, it takes only a few weeks for you to lose your level of fitness. In fact, many top athletes feel that even after only two or three days lay-off they begin to lose condition. The longer you lay off, the harder it is to get back to peak fitness.

There are different methods which allow you to assess and develop the components of fitness.

# Cardio-vascular endurance

## Assessing your level

We use heartbeat as a measure of cardio-vascular endurance. To assess your level of cardio-vascular endurance, you measure what happens to your heartbeat during exercise and how quickly it drops back to normal. Heartbeat is affected by your fitness, your age, your sex and, of course, your activity at the moment. The lower your heartbeat and the quicker your recovery, the fitter you are.

Two tests used to measure cardio-vascular endurance are:
- the Cooper 12-minute run test
- the Kasch–Boyer step test.

## The Cooper 12-minute run test

This test involves running as far as possible in 12 minutes. The further you can run, the higher your level of cardio-vascular endurance. You should do this test on a 400-metre track that has been measured out in 20-metre intervals. (See table 4.1.)

**Table 4.1:** Rating chart for the 12-minute run (distance in metres)

|  | Excellent | Good | Fair | Poor |
|---|---|---|---|---|
| **13–14 years** | | | | |
| Men | 2700 | 2400 | 2200 | 2100 |
| Women | 2000 | 1900 | 1600 | 1500 |
| **15–16 years** | | | | |
| Men | 2800 | 2500 | 2300 | 2200 |
| Women | 2100 | 1900 | 1700 | 1500 |
| **17–20 years** | | | | |
| Men | 3000 | 2700 | 2500 | 2300 |
| Women | 2300 | 2100 | 1800 | 1500 |

*The 1.6 km run test*
You can measure you cardio-vascular fitness against that of your age group by running 1.6 kilometres and checking your time.

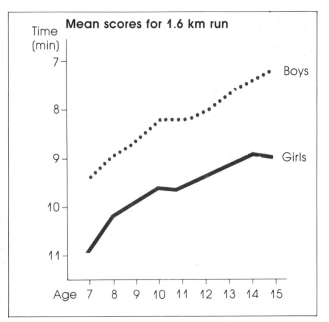

**Figure 4.1:** This graph shows the average performance of different age groups.

## The Kasch-Boyer step test

The step test is a simple test requiring a bench or chair 30 centimetres high. You step on to the bench with both feet and step down again at a pace of once every two seconds for three minutes.

Five seconds after the exercise, your pulse rate is taken for one minute. The lower your pulse rate, the higher your level of cardiovascular endurance.

**Table 4.2:** Rating chart for the step test in beats per minute

| Years | Excellent | Good | Fair | Poor |
|---|---|---|---|---|
| **13-14** | | | | |
| Men | 90 or less | 91–98 | 99–120 | 120 up |
| Women | 100 or less | 101–110 | 111–130 | 130 up |
| **15-16** | | | | |
| Men | 85 or less | 86–95 | 96–115 | 115 up |
| Women | 95 or less | 96–105 | 106–125 | 125 up |
| **17-20** | | | | |
| Men | 80 or less | 81–90 | 91–110 | 110 up |
| Women | 90 or less | 91–100 | 101–120 | 120 up |

Once you have worked out your cardiovascular endurance level, you can devise a programme to improve or maintain it. You can monitor improvement by repeating the tests once a month.

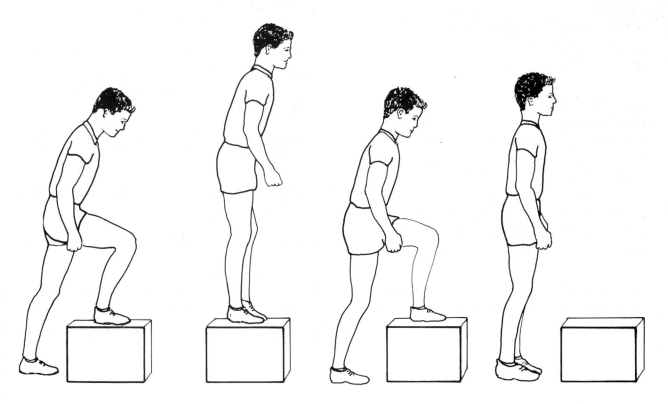

**Figure 4.2:** The Kasch–Boyer step test.

# Activities to improve cardio-vascular endurance

The best way to improve your cardio-vascular endurance is to work on two types of exercise:

- *Aerobic exercises.* In these exercises, your cardio-respiratory system feeds the muscles with oxygen to help produce energy. Aerobic exercises should be steady and extended. Examples of good aerobic exercise are brisk walking, jogging, swimming, aerobic dancing, cycling and vigorous sports.
- *Anaerobic exercises* are those which use energy produced without oxygen. They are short, intense exercises which often cause you to gasp. There must be rest periods between them and they should not be attempted by beginners or people with low cardio-vascular endurance. The exercises include fast sprints in running, swimming and cycling.

Aerobic and anaerobic exercises all increase your heartbeat and affect the cardio-respiratory system. To be safe, you must know the intensity, duration and frequency of the exercises suitable for your level of fitness. This can be worked out from your heartbeat. The starting point is your pulse at rest. To work out your pulse rate, rest for at least 15 minutes and then take your pulse for one minute. Then look at table 4.3 which shows you the heart rate which you should train at during exercise.

Two minutes after beginning an aerobic exercise, you should check your heartbeat again. In the case of anaerobic activity, take your pulse immediately after the exercise. This is done by counting your pulse for 15 seconds and multiplying it by 4. If your heartbeat is higher than desired, you should decrease the intensity of your exercise. If it is lower than desired, you can increase the intensity of exercise.

To improve your performance you should exercise at the desired level for 15 minutes at least three times a week. It is important to have at least one day per week off.

**Table 4.3:** Heart rate for exercising

| Resting heart rate per minute | Desired heart rate during aerobic exercise | | Desired heart rate during anaerobic exercise (not for beginners) |
|---|---|---|---|
| | **Beginner** | **Advanced** | |
| Below 50 | 135–140 | 145–150 | 165–170 |
| 51–70 | 141–145 | 151–155 | 171–175 |
| 71 and over | 146–150 | 156–160 | 176–180 |

*Source:* Charles B. Corbin and Ruth Lindsey, *Fitness for Life,* 2nd ed. (Glenview, Ill.: Scott, Foresman, 1983).

**Table 4.4:** Training schedule for cardio-vascular fitness

| | **How hard?** | **How long?** | **How often?** |
|---|---|---|---|
| **Aerobic** | Refer to heart rate table. Raise your heart rate to correct level. | For at least 15 minutes, preferably more. | At least 3 days per week, preferably more. |
| **Anaerobic** | Raise your heart rate to correct level. | 20 seconds, then jog slowly for 1 minute. Repeat this for at least 15 minutes. | At least 3 days per week, preferably more. |

*Source:* Adapted from Corbin and Lindsey, *Fitness for Life,* and from *Australia Sport: A Profile* (Canberra: AGPS, 1985).

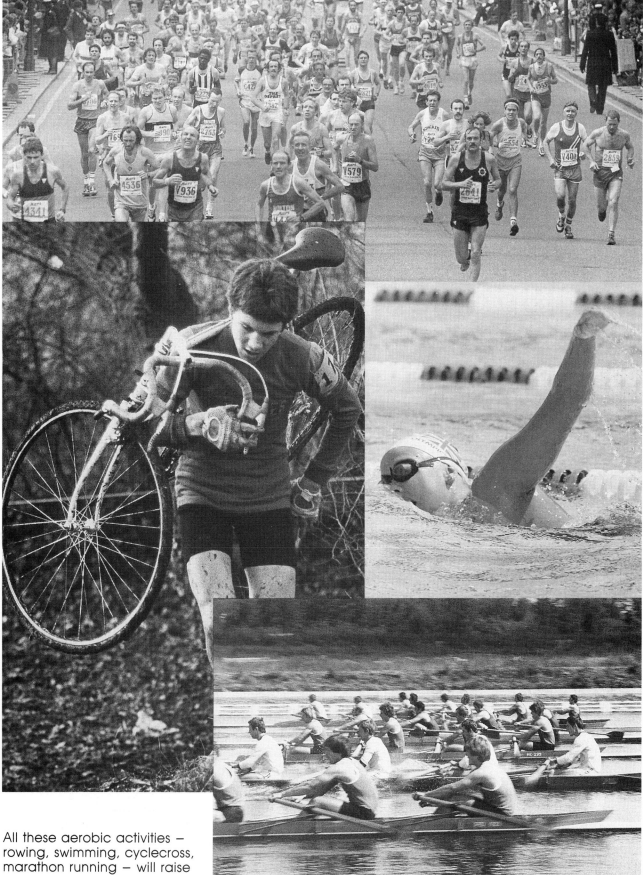

All these aerobic activities –
rowing, swimming, cyclecross,
marathon running – will raise
your heart rate.

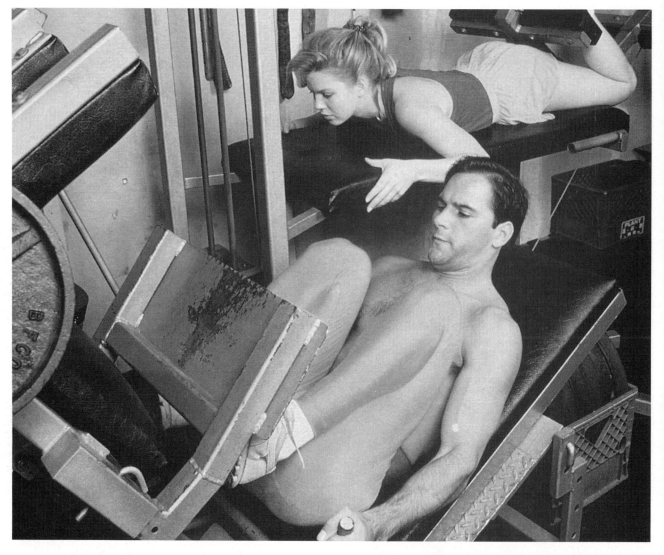

Science and technology play their part in helping to improve performance.

## Muscular endurance

Assessing muscular endurance by referring to a set table showing numbers of repetitions of exercises is not useful because body types are different. It is better to work individually. To assess your own muscular endurance, you must see how many repetitions of an exercise you can do comfortably. This will be your base level. To improve your level, work on increasing the number of repetitions. Remember, being able to do an exercise once, such as a push-up, requires strength; being able to do repetitions of push-ups requires endurance. The graphs in figure 4.3 show average performances of children in sit-ups and push-ups. and figures 4.4(a) to (f) illustrate exercises for specific muscles.

## Oxygen debt

When anaerobic exercise is performed, lactic acid is produced. Normally, this is broken down by oxygen to produce more energy. However, if there is not enough oxygen available, lactic acid builds up, and this lessens the ability of the muscles to contract, thus causing pain. The body will try to provide more oxygen by increasing the heartbeat and breathing rate, often through gasping and panting.

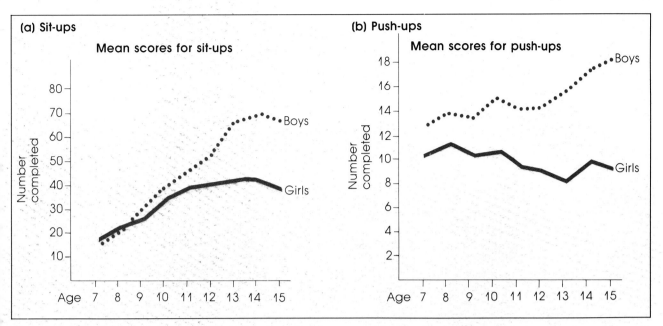

**Figure 4.3:** These graphs show the average performances of children in sit-ups and push-ups.

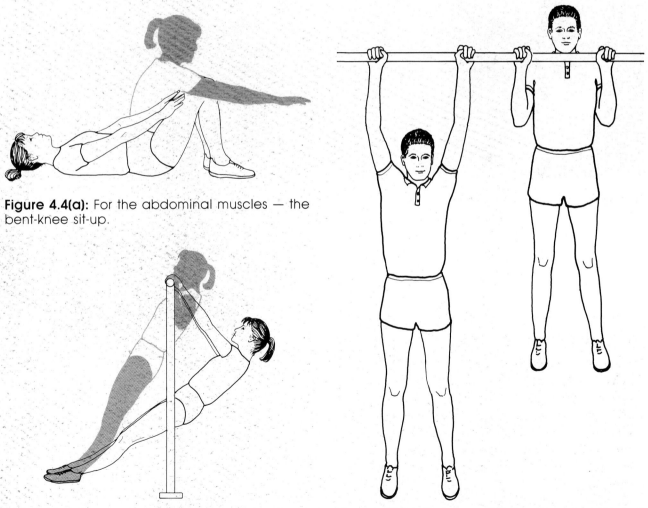

**Figure 4.4(a):** For the abdominal muscles — the bent-knee sit-up.

**Figure 4.4(b):** For arm and shoulder muscles — modified chin-ups (recommended for girls).

**Figure 4.4(c):** For arm and shoulder muscles — chin-ups.

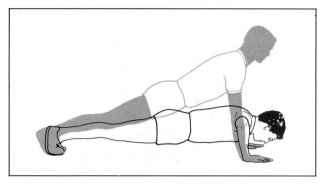

**Figure 4.4(d):** For the back of the arm (triceps), chest (pectoral) and shoulder (deltoid) muscles — push-ups. Medical authorities recommend that girls should do modified push-ups from the knees.

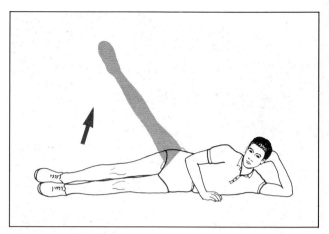

**Figure 4.4(e):** For hip muscles — side leg raises.

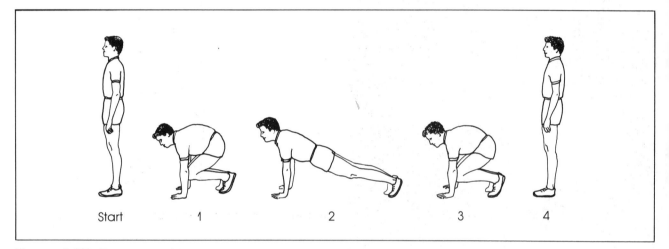

Start    1    2    3    4

**Figure 4.4(f):** For general leg, arm and body muscles — burpees.

# Strength

It is difficult to measure strength precisely without machines; therefore, this section will concentrate on methods of improving strength. Muscular strength is directly related to muscular endurance. As you improve your muscular endurance, your muscles will also strengthen. However, you can strengthen your muscles without having to do a large number of repetitions. Muscular strength increases when you overload the muscle with increased resistances in a training programme.

There are two ways to improve your strength:
● Isotonics — exercises with movement
● Isometrics — exercises without movement.

## Isotonics

There are some authorities who believe that weight training should not begin until the body is fully grown. If you are still growing, you should discuss weight training with your doctor before attempting it.

A weight training programme should overload the major muscle groups in the legs, chest, shoulders, arms, abdomen and back. You should begin with weights that are easy to lift and gradually, over a number of sessions, increase the weight so that the muscles are overloaded. It is a good idea to alternate exercises so that different muscles are overloaded. For instance, do one set of exercises that work the leg muscles, then another set that work the shoulder muscles, then back to the leg muscle exercises.

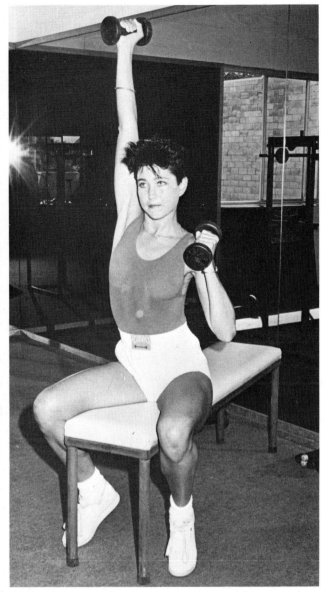

A variation of the standing press using dumbbells.

## Sample programme for general strength

The following programme takes approximately 30 minutes. Each exercise is done in three sets of ten repetitions, alternating with another exercise. For example, begin with 10 standing presses, then do 10 upright rowing exercises; repeat this sequence twice more. Then move on to the biceps curl and sit-ups sequence, doing 10 repetitions of one and then the other. Repeat this sequence twice more.

1. Standing press, figure 4.5(a), and
2. Upright rowing, figure 4.5(b).

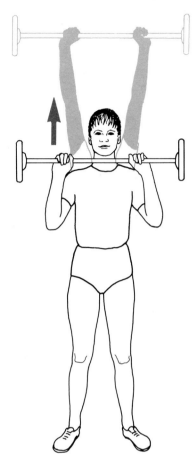

**Figure 4.5(a):** Standing press.

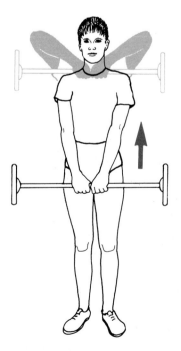

**Figure 4.5(b):** Upright rowing.

3. Biceps curl, figure 4.5(c),
   and
4. Sit-ups with weight held on chest.

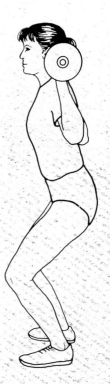

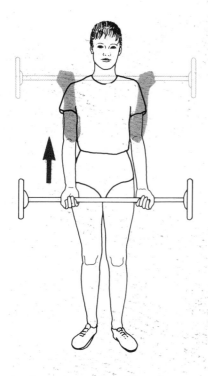

**Figure 4.5(e):** Half squats.

**Figure 4.5(c):** Biceps curl.

7. Heel lifts, figure 4.5(f).

5. Bench press, figure 4.5(d),
   and
6. Half squats, figure 4.5(e).

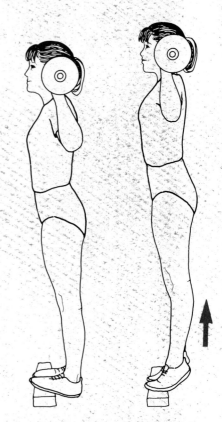

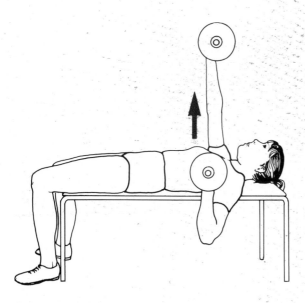

**Figure 4.5(d):** Bench press.

**Figure 4.5(f):** Heel lifts.

A programme like this carried out three times a week usually results in a significant increase in strength in about two months. Increasing the number of repetitions and decreasing the weights increases endurance.

To increase your strength without weights, you can do the exercises mentioned under muscular endurance (pp. 73–74). Begin with three sets of five for each exercise and gradually build up to three sets of ten.

## Isometrics

Muscle strength can also be developed through isometric exercises. These can be done almost anywhere and at any time. Any pressing or pulling against an immoveable object, thereby contracting your muscles, is an isometric exercise.

### Rules for isometric exercise

- People with heart problems or those who have been inactive for a long time should not do isometric exercises as blood circulation may slow down.
- Muscle contraction must be held for at least 5 seconds to be effective. Any more than 10 seconds is unnecessary.
- Contractions should be done at least twice.

- Do not hold your breath during contractions as this increases blood pressure and may cut off supply of blood to your brain.

## Flexibility

Flexibility is an important component of fitness because it often determines how well an athlete can perform. You may have a high level of endurance and a high level of strength, but if your muscles are tight and the joints inflexible your speed, agility, balance and range of movement could be decreased. You will also be more prone to muscle soreness and injury.

### Assessing flexibility

There are three common tests you can do under the supervision of a trained instructor to assess the flexibility of your body.

### Sit and reach test

The sit and reach test measures your ability to stretch the muscles of the lower back and the back of the legs (hamstrings). Sit on the floor with legs straight and feet flat against a base. Reach as far as possible towards your toes and hold for 3 seconds (see figure 4.6, p. 78).

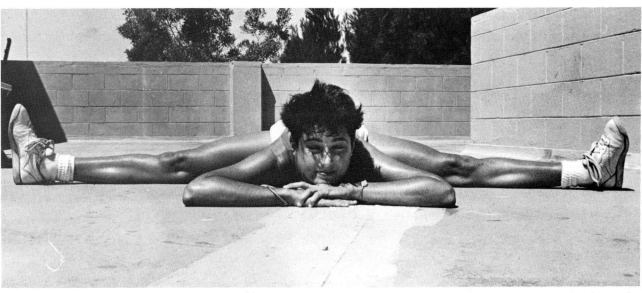

Flexibility like this comes only after many hours of flexibility exercises.

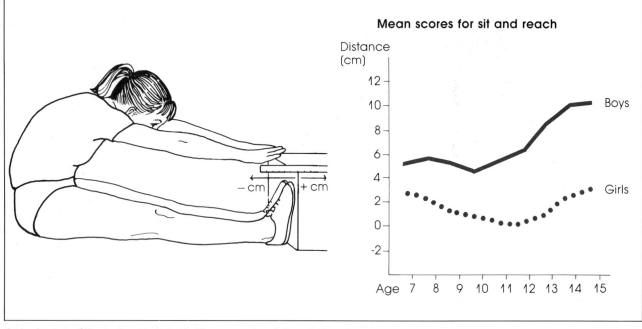

**Figure 4.6:** Sit and reach test. The graph at the right shows average performances of children in the sit and reach test.

## Arm and shoulder reach

This exercise measures your ability to stretch the muscles of the shoulders. Lie face down on the floor with arms straight. Hold a stick with your hands shoulder-width apart, raise your arms as high as possible and hold for 3 seconds. Keep your chin on the floor during the stretch (see figure 4.7).

## Trunk extension test

This test measures your ability to stretch the muscles of the upper back. Lie face down on the floor, put your hands behind your head and raise your head and shoulders as high as possible holding for 3 seconds (see figure 4.8).

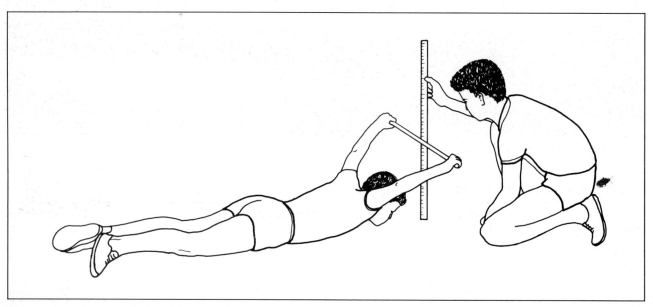

**Figure 4.7:** Arm and shoulder reach.

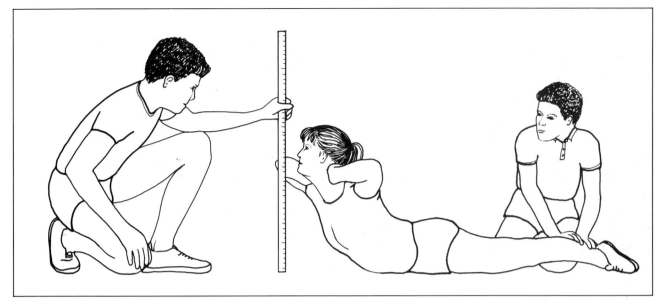

**Figure 4.8:** Trunk extension test.

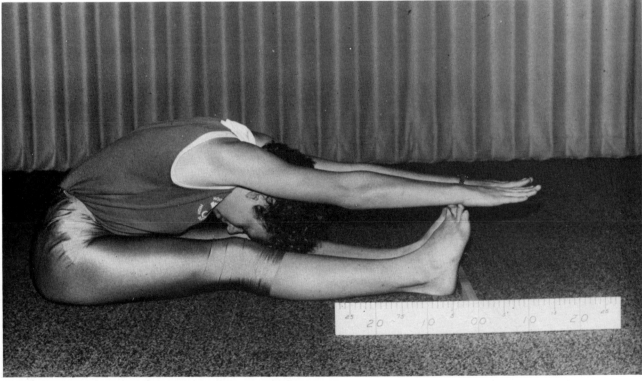

Flexibility is important for performance in many events.

**Table 4.5:** Flexibility rating table (in cm)

| Rating | Sit and reach (from fingers past toes) | Arm and shoulder reach (from floor to stick) | Trunk extension (from floor to chin) |
|---|---|---|---|
| Excellent | 25 | 35 | 55 |
| Good | 15 | 25 | 45 |
| Fair | −5 | 20 | 35 |
| Poor | −15 | 15 | 30 |

*Source:* Adapted from Corbin and Lindsay, *Fitness for Life.*

# How to improve your flexibility

When you start a stretching programme, remember the following points:

- Unless you are a highly trained athlete, avoid bouncy, jerky movements as they can cause tearing of muscles, ligaments and tendons.
- Do stretching exercises for the specific muscles used in the sport you play. General stretching is a worthwhile addition.
- Flexibility exercises should be done at least three times a week.
- Flexibility should be within the normal range of movement to prevent injury.

The exercises in figure 4.9(a) to (i) will stretch all the major muscle groups of the body and will increase your flexibility. You should aim to do twenty of each.

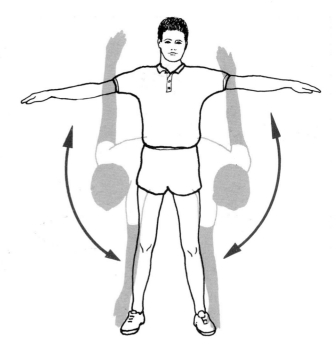

**Figure 4.9(b):** Windmills.

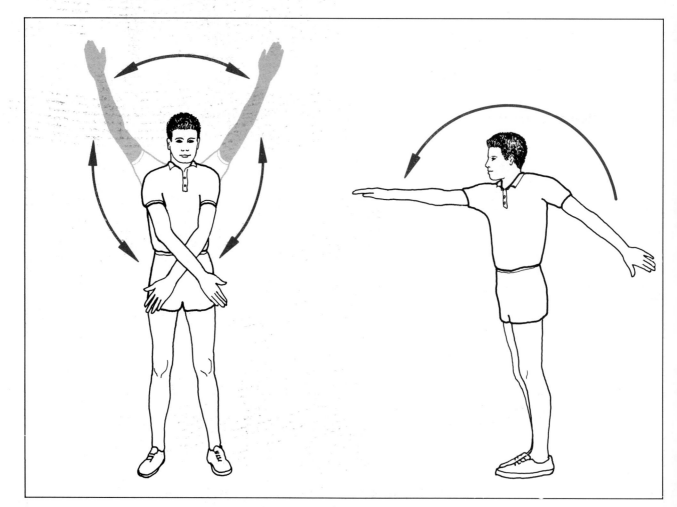

**Figure 4.9(a):** Arm circles.

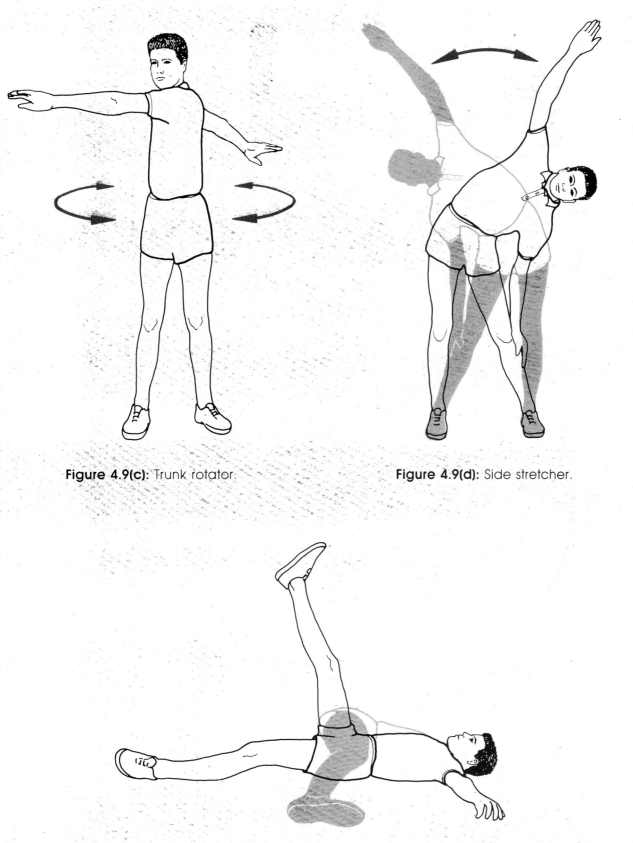

**Figure 4.9(c):** Trunk rotator.

**Figure 4.9(d):** Side stretcher.

**Figure 4.9(e):** Sideways leg stretch.

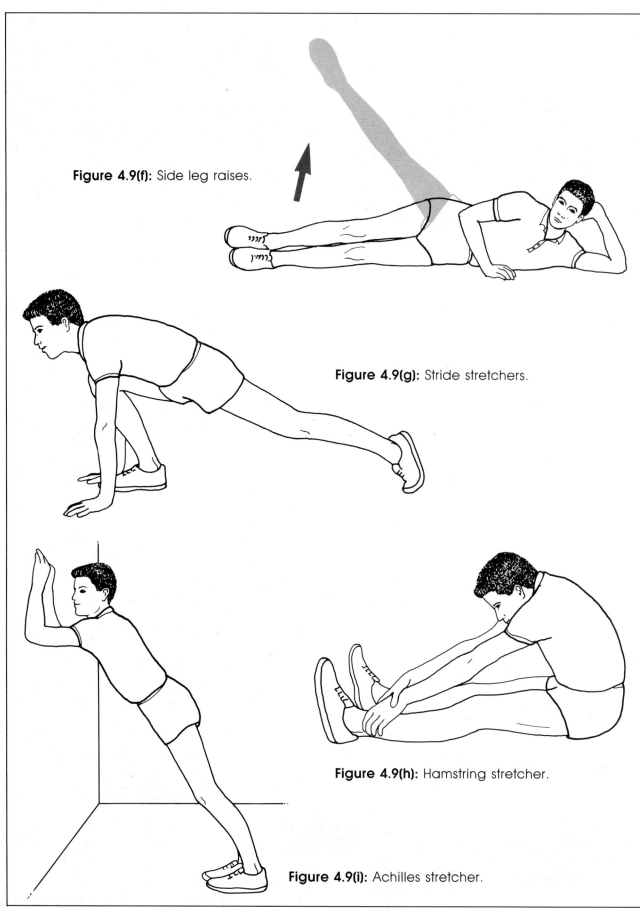

**Figure 4.9(f):** Side leg raises.

**Figure 4.9(g):** Stride stretchers.

**Figure 4.9(h):** Hamstring stretcher.

**Figure 4.9(i):** Achilles stretcher.

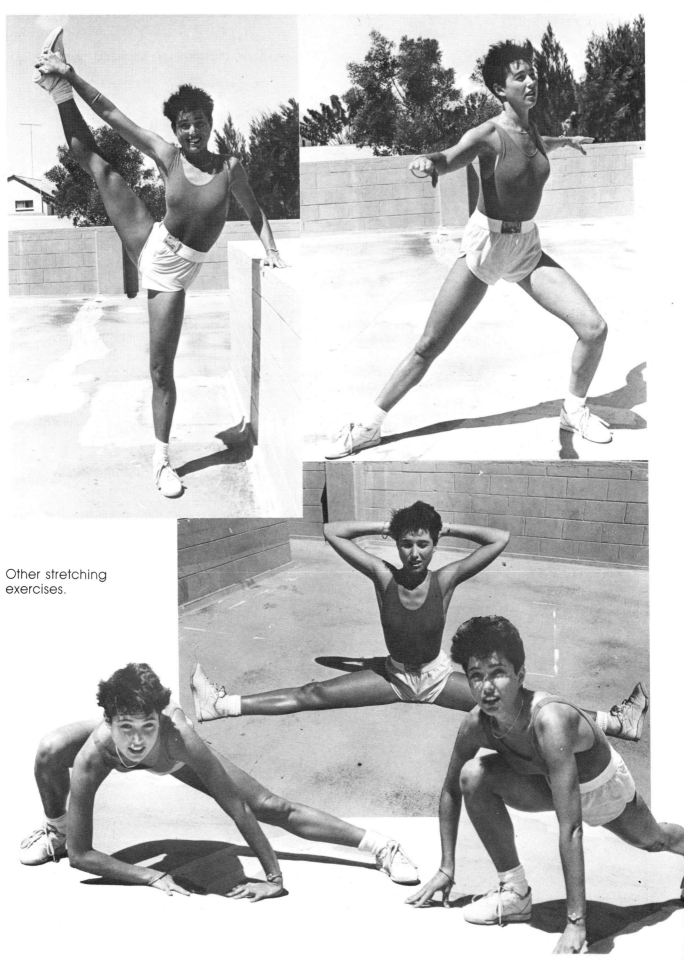

Other stretching
exercises.

# Power

Power is used in sports where explosive strength is required. A runner or swimmer at the start needs power; shot-putters and discus and javelin throwers all need power; golfers, tennis players and cricketers all use power when hitting the ball. Muscle power depends on two factors: speed and strength.

To assess your level of leg muscle power, there is an easy test to perform – the standing long jump.

**Table 4.6:** Rating chart for power in standing long jump (metres)

| Rating | Male | Female |
|---|---|---|
| Excellent | 2.10 | 1.85 |
| Good | 2.00 | 1.65 |
| Fair | 1.75 | 1.45 |
| Poor | 1.50 | 1.30 |

*Source:* Adapted from Corbin and Lindsey, *Fitness for Life.*

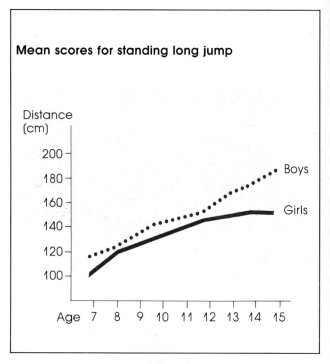

Mean scores for standing long jump

**Figure 4.10:** Average performances of children in the standing long jump.

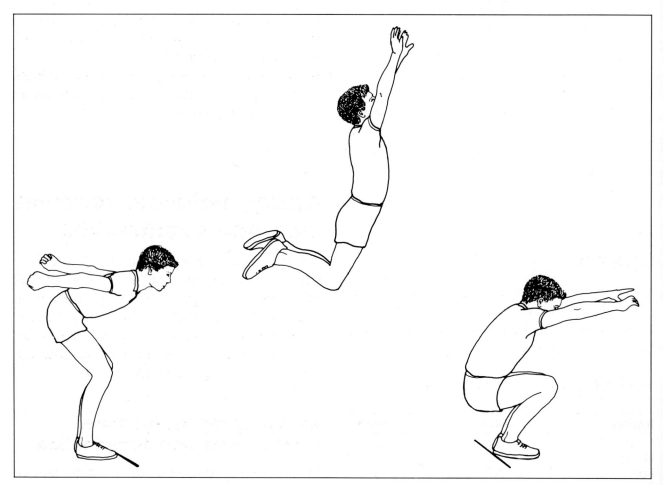

**Figure 4.11:** The standing long jump.

Power can be improved by doing exercises to increase both your strength and your speed.

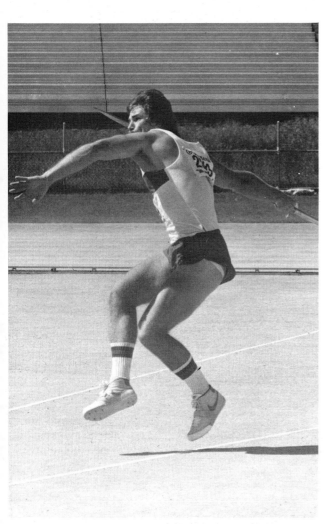

Using power.

# Speed

Speed depends on how quickly you can contract your muscles. To assess your whole body's speed, measure how long it takes you to run 50 metres.

**Table 4.7:** Rating chart for 50-metre sprint (in seconds)

| Rating | Male | Female |
|---|---|---|
| Excellent | 7.0 | 8.0 |
| Good | 7.5 | 8.5 |
| Fair | 8.0 | 9.0 |
| Poor | 8.5 | 9.5 |

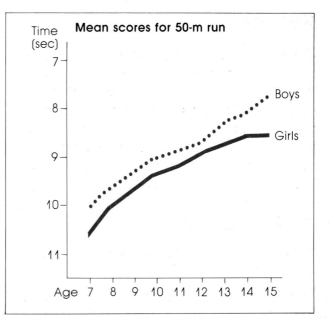

**Figure 4.12:** Average performances of children in the 50-metre run.

Your speed can be improved in three ways:
- by increasing the strength of muscles
- by improving your style so that any bad habits are corrected
- by using a training programme which includes lots of speed work and occurs at least three times a week.

# Agility, balance, reaction time and coordination

Agility, balance, reaction time and coordination are components of fitness that are all skill-related, and your level of performance often depends on your natural ability. People who naturally have a high level of one or more of these components tend to take up sports which require them.

## Assessing agility, balance, reaction time and coordination

The following tests can be used to assess your ability in these four components.

## Test for agility — the Illinois agility run

Lie face down with your forehead on the starting line and your hands beside your chest. As soon as the starting signal is given, jump up and follow the zig-zag pattern as shown in figure 4.13. Try to complete the course as quickly as possible.

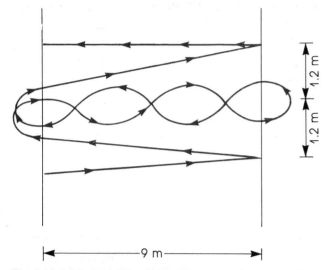

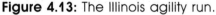

**Figure 4.13:** The Illinois agility run.

**Table 4.8:** Rating chart for Illinois agility run (in seconds)

| Rating | Male | Female |
|--------|------|--------|
| Excellent | 15.0–15.6 | 18.4–19.1 |
| Good | 16.3–17.2 | 19.8–20.8 |
| Average | 17.6 | 21.2 |
| Poor | 18.0–18.9 | 21.6–22.5 |

## Test for balance — the stork stand

Stand comfortably on both feet and place your hands on your hips. Lift one leg and place the toes against the knee of the other leg (see figure 4.14). When the signal is given, raise your heel and stand on your toes, balancing for as long as possible without your heel touching the floor or the other foot moving away from your knee.

**Table 4.9:** Rating chart for the stork stand

| Rating | Seconds |
|--------|---------|
| Excellent | 60 |
| Good | 40 |
| Fair | 25 |
| Poor | 10 |

**Figure 4.14** The stork stand.

## Test for reaction time

This test needs to be done in pairs.

*Step 1.* Have your partner hold the top of a 1-metre ruler at the 1-centimetre mark. Your partner should hold the ruler vertically, but you should not touch it.

*Step 2.* Place your thumb and fingers at the 60-centimetre mark without touching the ruler. Your arm should rest on the edge of a table with only your hand extending over the edge.

*Step 3.* When your partner drops the ruler without warning, catch it as quickly as possible between thumb and fingers.

**Table 4.10:** Rating chart for reaction time

| Rating | Position on ruler |
|--------|-------------------|
| Excellent | 52-cm mark |
| Good | 45-cm mark |
| Fair | 35-cm mark |
| Poor | below the 35-cm mark |

*Source:* Adapted from Corbin and Lindsey, *Fitness for Life.*

## Test for coordination — alternate hand wall throw

Stand 2 metres away from and facing a wall. At the starting signal, throw a ball underarm against the wall with your right hand and catch it in your left hand. Then throw it with your left hand and catch it with your right. Do this as quickly as possible for 30 seconds.

**Table 4.11:** Rating chart for alternate hand wall throw

| Rating | Male | Female |
|---|---|---|
| Excellent | 36 | 27 |
| Good | 30 | 21 |
| Average | 28 | 19 |
| Poor | 23 | 14 |

## How to improve your agility, balance, reaction time and coordination

Repeated practice is the only way to improve these components.

- Agility – move your body quickly in different directions.
- Balance – walk along a line or a narrow beam.
- Reaction time – practise starts, stopping penalty goals, catching objects unexpectedly.
- Coordination – practise goal-shooting, ball-throwing or any other hand–eye or foot–eye coordination skills over and over.

**Table 4.12:** Physical activities and components for fitness

| Sport or activity | Develops cardio-vascular endurance | Develops muscular endurance | Develops strength | Develops flexibility | Power | Speed | Agility | Balance | Reaction time | Coordination |
|---|---|---|---|---|---|---|---|---|---|---|
| American football | Excellent | Good | Good | Fair | Excellent | Excellent | Excellent | Good | Excellent | Good |
| Archery | Poor | Poor | Fair | Poor | Poor | Poor | Poor | Fair | Poor | Excellent |
| Badminton | Fair | Fair | Poor | Fair | Fair | Good | Good | Good | Good | Excellent |
| Basketball | Excellent | Fair | Poor | Poor | Excellent | Good | Excellent | Good | Excellent | Excellent |
| Bowling | Poor | Poor | Poor | Poor | Fair | Fair | Fair | Good | Poor | Excellent |
| Cycling | Excellent | Good | Good | Poor | Poor | Fair | Poor | Excellent | Fair | Fair |
| Dance, aerobic | Excellent | Good | Fair | Good | Poor | Poor | Good | Fair | Fair | Good |
| Fencing | Fair | Good | Fair | Fair | Good | Excellent | Good | Good | Excellent | Excellent |
| Football | Excellent | Good | Fair | Fair | Good | Good | Excellent | Fair | Good | Excellent |
| Golf (walking) | Fair | Poor | Poor | Fair | Good | Poor | Fair | Fair | Poor | Excellent |
| Gymnastics | Fair | Excellent | Excellent | Excellent | Excellent | Fair | Excellent | Excellent | Good | Excellent |
| Hiking | Good | Excellent | Fair | Fair | Fair | Poor | Fair | Fair | Poor | Fair |
| Horseriding | Poor | Poor | Poor | Poor | Poor | Poor | Good | Good | Fair | Good |
| Jogging | Excellent | Good | Poor | Poor | Poor | Poor | Poor | Fair | Poor | Fair |
| Judo/karate | Poor | Fair | Fair | Fair | Excellent | Excellent | Excellent | Good | Excellent | Excellent |
| Pool/billiards | Poor | Poor | Poor | Poor | Fair | Poor | Fair | Fair | Poor | Good |
| Rowing, crew | Excellent | Excellent | Fair | Poor | Excellent | Fair | Good | Fair | Poor | Excellent |
| Sailing | Poor | Poor | Poor | Poor | Fair | Poor | Good | Good | Good | Good |
| Skating | Fair-good | Fair | Poor | Poor | Fair | Good | Good | Excellent | Poor | Good |
| Skiing, cross-country | Excellent | Good | Fair | Poor | Excellent | Fair | Good | Fair | Poor | Excellent |
| Skiing, downhill | Poor | Fair | Fair | Poor | Good | Poor | Excellent | Excellent | Good | Excellent |
| Swimming | Excellent | Good | Fair | Fair | Fair | Poor | Good | Fair | Poor | Good |
| Table tennis | Poor | Poor | Poor | Poor | Fair | Fair | Fair | Fair | Good | Good |
| Tennis | Fair-good | Fair | Poor | Poor | Good | Good | Good | Poor | Good | Excellent |
| Volleyball | Fair | Poor | Fair | Poor | Fair | Fair | Good | Fair | Good | Excellent |
| Walking | Fair | Fair | Poor | Poor | Poor | Poor | Poor | Poor | Poor | Poor |
| Waterskiing | Fair | Fair | Fair | Poor | Fair | Fair | Good | Good | Poor | Good |
| Weight training | Poor | Excellent | Excellent | Poor | Fair | Poor | Poor | Fair | Poor | Fair |

*Source:* Adapted from Corbin and Lindsey, *Fitness for Life.*

# Training for performance

In the previous section, you have seen how you can measure and improve individual components of fitness. However, many people want to be able to plan training sessions. Before you plan a training programme, it is a good idea to have a check-up and chat with your doctor, even if you are young and feel healthy. This is absolutely essential for anyone in their mid-thirties or older who has not been actively exercising.

Whether you are a beginner or more advanced in exercising, all training sessions should be divided into three parts:

- the warm-up
- the training activities
- the cool-down.

## The warm-up

The warm-up is important because:

- it prepares the muscles for vigorous action
- it prepares the cardio-vascular system for vigorous action
- it prepares the joints by warming the synovial fluid
- it prepares the individual psychologically for the activities.

Warming up increases the blood supply to the muscles and raises their temperature. This makes them more flexible and less likely to be injured. A warm-up should be done in two stages:

- stretching stage
- muscle warm-up.

### The stretching stage

Stretching exercises should be done carefully to reduce risk of injury to the muscles or joints. Concentrate on the muscles and joints you will need to use during your training activities. Usually, 10 minutes of stretching exercises is enough.

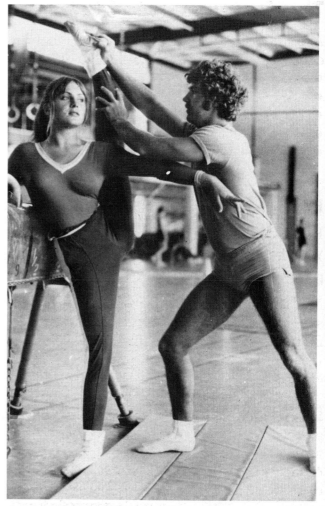

A gymnast warming up. The warm-up and cool-down are just as important before and after competition as before and after training activities. Most world-class athletes spend at least 30 minutes doing stretching exercises before a major event.

### Muscle warm-up

Once your stretching exercises are completed, you are ready to begin warming up the muscles. This must be done slowly to avoid injury. The best way to warm up muscles is to perform with less intensity the movements you will be doing during the training activities; for example, a runner should jog slowly, gradually building up speed; footballers should jog and handle or kick the ball; tennis players should rally. Once the muscles are warmed up, you can extend yourself to full speed and strength.

# The training activities

Activities for a training session should be chosen using the following principles:
- background
- specificity
- overloading
- hard days and easy days
- peaking.

## Background

Exercises should be chosen according to your level of fitness.

### Beginners

Many beginners are impatient and want to start a vigorous training programme on the first day. This increases the risk of injury. Beginners should start with moderate exercise.

Exercise should be sufficient to cause heavy breathing but not so hard as to cause gasping and breathlessness. A good rule of thumb for beginners is that, while exercising, they should still be able to hum a tune or carry on a conversation. The length of the activities should not exceed 15–20 minutes at a steady pace until the beginner feels comfortable in increasing the load. Exercise should be undertaken three to five times a week. A beginner's programme should last about one month.

### Pre-season build-up

It is important to begin your programme slowly and not to strain yourself, especially if you have been inactive for a long period because of injury or lay-off. Laying a foundation and gradually increasing the workload will improve your fitness safely and without strain.

## Specificity

Your training activities must include:
- exercises to improve the particular component of fitness which applies to your sport; for example, strength for weightlifters, endurance for marathon runners, flexibility for gymnasts.

- exercises to improve the muscle group most important to your performance; for example, shoulder and leg muscles for rowers, arm muscles for tennis players, leg muscles for skiers.

- activities to improve the skills of your sport; for example, dribbling in hockey, goal-shooting in netball, bowling or batting in cricket, serving in tennis, driving and putting in golf.

## Overloading

In order to make progress through training you need to use the principle of overloading to improve your aerobic activity, muscular strength and flexibility. This means that those body systems have to work harder than normal. You can do this in three ways:
- by working harder, running faster, lifting heavier weights, stretching further so that you increase the **intensity** of exercise
- by training more often and increasing the **frequency** of exercise
- by training for longer periods of time and increasing the **duration** of exercise.

## Hard days and easy days

Hard days are days on which you carry out a vigorous training session. Because hard training breaks down muscle tissue, it is important to allow rest time for the muscles to recover. Therefore, a hard day should be followed by an easy day of exercise on which the muscles are not overloaded. By the next hard day, the muscles will be stronger and endurance will have increased. There should be no more than three hard days per week.

# Peaking

Peaking is the method by which highly trained athletes can achieve their maximum or peak performance at a particular competition. Peaking allows the athlete to avoid fatigue and staleness. The timing and method of peaking in a training programme depends on the sport involved. However, to peak, an athlete normally:

- decreases the length of a training session
- decreases the frequency of exercises in a session
- increases the intensity of anaerobic training.

# Choosing training activities

- Choose exercises to develop the components of fitness important to you.
- Choose the skills important to your sport and allocate practice time to them.
- Vary your sessions according to your needs. You may want to develop a gym programme in consultation with an instructor; you may want to train with a group or alone; you may want to include one or more of the following methods:
  - continuous training
  - interval training
  - circuit training
  - Fartlek training.

## Continuous training

This method of training means you continue training at generally the same pace for at least 30 minutes. At the beginning of a fitness programme, you may find this difficult, but as you gradually improve you will find it easier to maintain the same pace for a longer period. Continuous training can be used for sports requiring a high level of cardio-vascular fitness.

## Interval training

Interval training involves alternating short, near-maximum bursts of speed with periods of rest or mild exercise; for example, a swim-ming session could include ten 50-metre sprints with 15 seconds rest in between; in athletics, you could run five 400-metre sprints with a 400-metre slow jog in between each sprint.

The aim is to increase your ability to produce bursts of speed during competition. Even marathon runners undertake interval training as they know that, at some time during the race, they may have to accelerate to break up the field. Interval training causes more pain than continuous training because you have to perform at near-maximum level for periods of time. Activities which are suitable for interval training are running, swimming, cycling or rowing. Choose the one which helps your sport most. In interval training, the muscles must be overloaded in four different ways:

- by increasing the speed
- by decreasing the rest period
- by increasing the repetitions
- by increasing the distance.

The main benefit of interval training is that the anaerobic fitness level is increased in a way that could not be done with continuous training. An increase in anaerobic fitness results in an increase in sprinting ability.

## Circuit training

A circuit consists of a number of stations at each of which you perform a particular activity; it could be to run, exercise, use weights or practise a skill. The circuit is completed as quickly as possible. The main aim of circuit training is to build up cardio-vascular and muscular endurance, muscular strength, and flexibility. There are many benefits of circuit training:

- A variety of activities means that you are less likely to become bored.
- Each activity can be performed at near-maximum levels thereby increasing your anaerobic as well as aerobic fitness.
- You can work at your own pace.
- A circuit can be set up to suit you and can concentrate on any weakness you may have.

- A circuit can be set up almost anywhere, from out in the park, to a room in the house.

A circuit should consist of about eight to ten stations and take about 8–12 minutes to complete. The activities should be spaced so that the same muscle groups are not used consecutively. A rest of 2–3 minutes can be taken between each circuit.

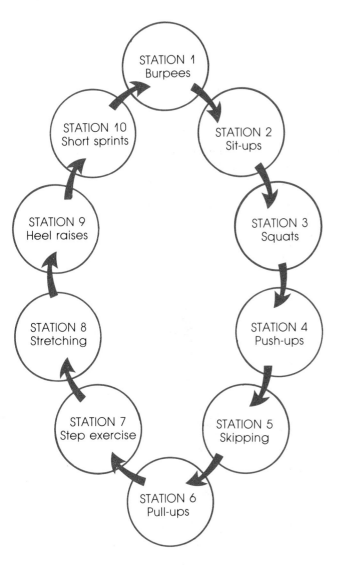

**Figure 4.15:** An endurance circuit.

### Fartlek training

This form of training was developed in Sweden and means "speed and play". Its aim is to run fast when you feel like it, jog when you get tired, and speed up again when you

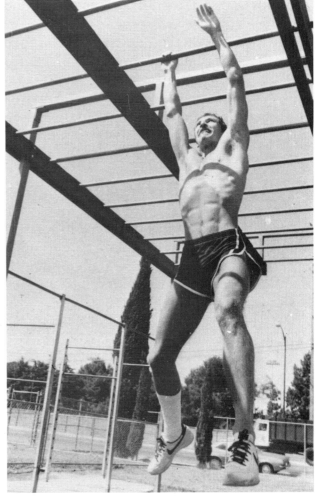

This is the kind of exercise that could be used in one station of a circuit.

recover. Although Fartlek is not as controlled as interval training, it still requires a strong will to be able to perform at near-maximum effort several times during a training session.

## The cool-down

All training sessions should finish with the cool-down. This is the tapering-off period after a hard, strenuous training session, and is as important as the warm-up. At the end of such a session, a large supply of blood remains in the muscles. If this is not returned quickly to the circulation, pooling of blood may occur in the muscles, a shortage of blood to the brain can result, and you could faint or collapse.

The best way to cool down is to continue the activity but at a much slower pace; for example, keep jogging or walking and gradually slow down until the heart returns to a steady rate. Muscle stretching should also be done during the cool-down stage.

# Food for fitness

Athletes who are heavily involved in sport or plan to start a heavy training programme need to be particularly careful about diet. A more detailed explanation of diet can be found in chapter 8.

## Water

Athletes lose fluid through sweating and increased breathing rate. Therefore, they must drink water during prolonged activity, otherwise they will suffer from dehydration.

## Protein

Protein is essential for developing muscles, bones, skin, tendons and all the organs of the body. A normal balanced diet contains sufficient protein. About 15 per cent of an athlete's diet should consist of protein. Excess protein is merely changed to fat or excreted.

## Carbohydrates

Carbohydrates are essential as they provide you with the energy needed to perform. Carbohydrates which are not used immediately are stored in the liver and muscles as glycogen. A good glycogen store is needed especially in endurance sports where the muscles have to work over long periods of time. The best source of carbohydrates for athletes is the complex carbohydrates in rice, pasta and potatoes. About 55 per cent of an athlete's diet should be carbohydrates.

# Hitting the wall

In long-distance endurance events, the athlete can lose all the glycogen from the muscles and there is no fuel left for the muscles. The athlete stops or at best staggers on painfully. When this happens it is called "hitting the wall" and can occur to any athlete if the muscles have been worked too hard or too fast. Only after renewing the glycogen by eating carbohydrates can the muscles work properly again. This takes time.

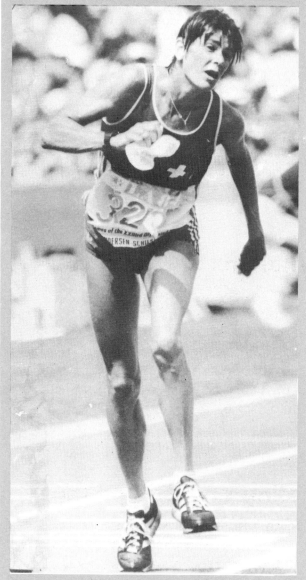

This Olympic marathon runner had "hit the wall" several kilometres earlier, and by continuing to run became dangerously dehydrated, overheated and exhausted by the time she finished the race.

# Carbohydrate loading

Carbohydrate loading is totally unnecessary in an event that lasts less than two hours of continuous exercise. It is sometimes used by endurance athletes to increase the normal amount of glycogen in the muscles, so that it is stored ready for use in competition. In the days before an event, such athletes eat large amounts of complex carbohydrates.

# Fats

Although fat is a concentrated form of energy, most athletes try to keep their fat intake to a minimum in order to keep their weight down.

# Vitamins and minerals

Vitamins and minerals are essential for good performance, but only small amounts are necessary, and these can be obtained from a normal diet. If, however, you feel constantly tired when you train, you should ask your doctor to look at your vitamin and mineral intake.

# Eating and competing

You should train and compete on an empty stomach. If you have food in your stomach, blood has to be pumped there for digestion to occur. When you begin using your muscles in competition, the blood flows away from the stomach to these muscles. The stomach muscles will then lack oxygen and cramping may result. The time it takes for your stomach to empty depends upon how fit you are, how you feel and what you eat. For the average person, it takes about 6 hours but for a highly fit athlete it takes only about 2 hours for food to pass through the stomach. On days when an important competition is being held and the athlete is keyed-up, it takes longer. Fats and protein take much longer to digest than carbohydrates.

# What to eat before competing

Your last meal before a match or competition should contain:
- very little protein or fat. They are not a source of immediate energy and the waste products from their breakdown can cause tiredness.
- plenty of complex carbohydrates but very little sugar. Pancakes, spaghetti, bread and fruit are high in complex carbohydrates and easily digestable. However, large amounts of sugar taken a few hours before competition will result in an upsurge in glucose levels followed by a dramatic drop as insulin clears it from the blood. This in turn will cause hunger and fatigue. A small amount of sugar immediately before your event will provide you with extra energy.
- plenty of fluid. Exercising causes a loss of fluid through breathing and sweating. When you lose 3 per cent of your body weight in fluid, your temperature rises and your muscles cannot contract properly. During a long endurance event such as a marathon, it is important to constantly replenish your supply of fluid. Do not wait until you are thirsty, because by then it is already too late.

# Fads and fallacies in fitness

There are many unusual techniques that people have used in an attempt to improve their performance. Many of these techniques are expensive, painful, inconvenient and even dangerous. Very few have proved to be successful. Be very careful about any "miracle" formula for increased performance.

- *Super doses of vitamins.* There is no scientific evidence that proves that taking vitamin tablets improves performance. In fact, overdoses of vitamins can be dangerous.
- *Weight-loss equipment.* Vibrating belts, rollers and muscle stimulators are just some of the machines advertised as getting rid of unwanted fat. They may massage you but they do *not* get rid of or "break down" fat.
- *Plastic or rubber sweatsuits.* These are sometimes worn during exercise and will certainly increase weight loss — but only in the immediate short term. The loss is only fluid, which will have to be replaced later. In fact, these suits can be dangerous if the user overheats.
- *Saunas.* As with the sweatsuit, the sauna makes you perspire, but you will have to replace the fluid later.
- *Fad diets.* A special diet may cause you to lose weight temporarily, but unless it is a well-balanced diet it will be harmful in the long term.
- *Spot reduction.* Exercising a particular muscle does not take fat from that muscle. Many people want to have thinner legs or smaller waists, but this cannot be achieved by simply doing leg or waist exercises. When weight is lost owing to diet or exercise, the weight is lost evenly from *all over the body.*

# 5

# Sports injuries and their prevention

The long hours of training involved in most sports and the demands of competition can sometimes lead to a number of injuries. We have all seen or read about competitors with blisters, sprains, strains, tears and the occasional broken bone. Injuries need time to repair depending on the extent of the injury.

When players are not training and playing, the level of their skills and fitness decreases.

Two or three weeks out of a sport means that a swimmer can lose the feel for the water, a footballer can be dropped from the team, and an athlete can miss an important competition.

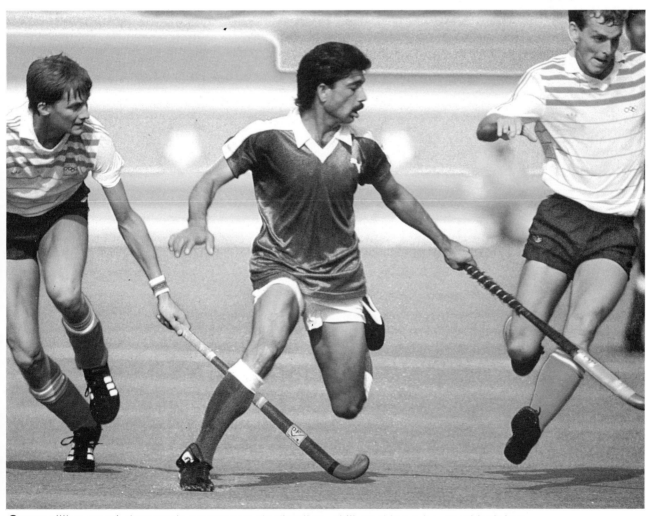

Competitive sport demands enormous dedication, skill and long hours of training.

Most importantly, the time lost during recovery from an injury can lead to a loss in performance and, if the injury is bad enough, this loss in performance may never be fully recovered.

In addition, injury causes pain, loss of fitness and mobility and, for the professional, loss of income.

For these reasons, this chapter:
- gives you an insight into the causes of sports injuries
- looks at types of sports injuries
- suggests methods of preventing injury or the worsening of injury.

This work is not intended to make you an expert in sports medicine. If you are unsure or the injury persists, you should always seek medical advice.

# The causes of sports injuries

The causes of sports injuries fall into two categories:
- external causes
- internal causes.

Below are many common causes of sports injuries in these groupings.

## External causes

Injuries occur when an outside force is applied to the victim:
- *body contact:* scrum, head-on collision, tackle
- *hit by an object:* racquet, stick, hard ball, bat

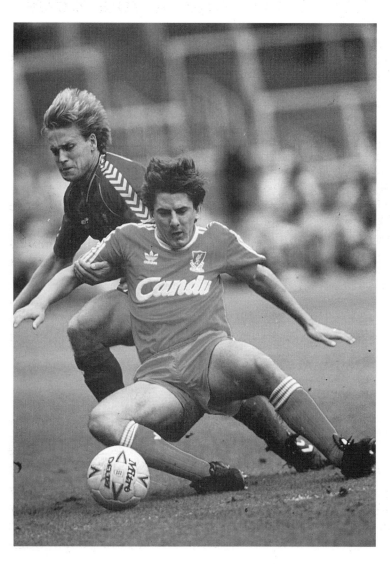

The crunch of a tackle can cause injury.

- *vehicular accident:* ski, car, hang-glider, boat, bicycle
- *environmental:* hit a wall, post or floor; fall on a hard track or pitch; wet or hard ground; weather conditions.

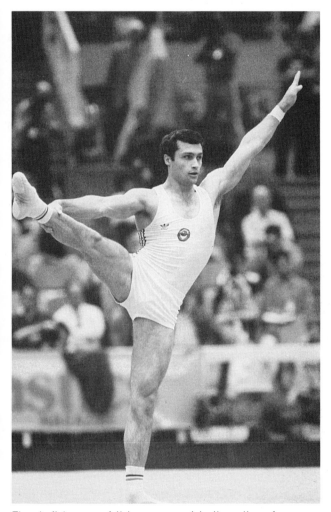

The left knee of this gymnast is the site of possible internal stress.

## Internal causes

Injuries can occur when stress develops within the athlete:

- *instant injury:* sudden tear of muscle; rupture of tendon or ligament; sprained joint
- *overuse:* inflammation of tendons, muscles, joints or bones resulting from long periods of overuse.

# Prevention of sports injuries

Before we look at specific injuries and their prevention, it is important to understand that there are general, commonsense factors that can be taken into account to avoid sports injuries. These factors include:

- knowledge of your body
- player suitability
- training methods
- protective equipment
- the rules of the game
- facilities.

## Knowledge of your body

Knowledge of how your body functions, how it moves, the forces that act on it during movement and the effects of training will provide you with an understanding of your body and its capabilities.

You can use this understanding to help you to prevent damage to your body when training and playing sport. This understanding is gained when you study:

- your body, its systems, and how these systems function
- your body in movement – biomechanics provides a sound scientific basis for movement in sports
- fitness for sport – this provides you with an insight into what you need to do in order to ensure you are fit to take part in sport.

## Player suitability

Understanding your own body helps you to select sports that are suited to your body type. It is obvious that people are physically different. It is also obvious that certain body types are more suited to some sports than others; for example, tall, lean people often

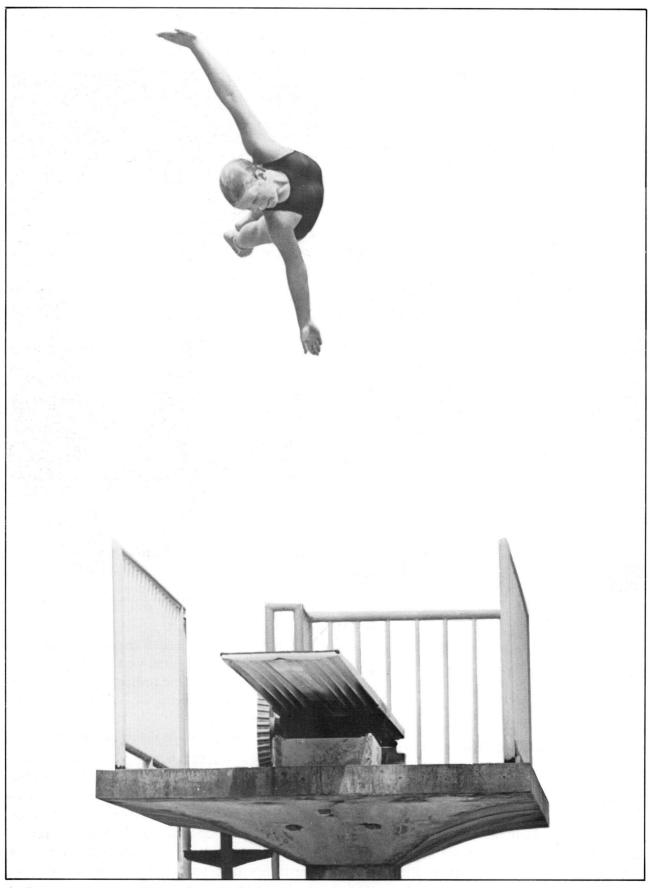

A diver needs a sound knowledge of how the body moves.

make better basketballers, heavier people do well in discus and shot-put, and thinner people are usually better performers in marathons. This does not mean that you should choose a sport simply because your body type seems to fit that sport. What it does mean, however, is that if you choose a sport for which your body type appears unsuited, you may have to train more to develop skills and to be fitter than other people in that sport.

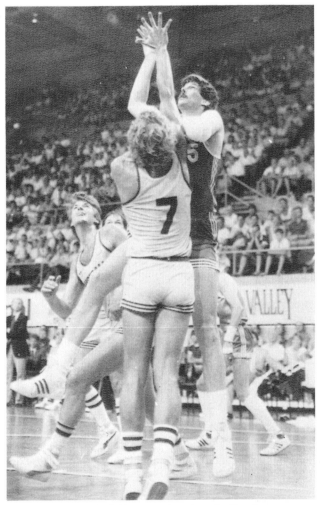

It helps to be tall if you play basketball.

# Training methods

Many experts feel that the most important factor in the prevention of injury is the development of a high level of skill and fitness. Athletes who are not fit, whose training is unsuitable or who play while not fully recovered from one injury are exposing themselves to risk of a serious injury.

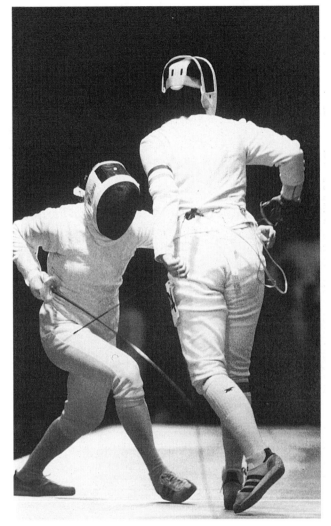

Competitors develop a high level of skill and fitness.

Pre-season fitness tests demanded by many clubs help you to assess your progress. Trainers and coaches often give players specific tasks based on these tests to strengthen the body, increase cardio-vascular fitness or improve flexibility.

Training should start well before the beginning of a sport's season to allow all the components of fitness to be fully developed. This allows a gradual increase in training load. To start sprints, use heavy weights or run and swim long distances in the second or third training session is likely to lead to further injury.

Too often, injuries are the result of training overload. Remember, continually sore muscles, bones or joints means something is wrong and you should seek professional help.

Tight, inflexible muscles cause too much strain and injury can occur. Always maintain an exercise programme that increases your flexibility even in the off-season and particularly before and after you compete.

# Protective equipment

Protective equipment in sport is any article that gives protection to the players. Thus, a well-fitting sports uniform and shoes are just as important as a helmet, mouthguard or body pads.

## Footwear

Good protective gear is often expensive, but it is designed to minimise the chance of injury. You should look for well-fitting shoes with firm, well-placed arch supports made from good material, and a sole suited to the type of playing surface and the sport you intend to play.

## Mouthguards

Mouthguards protect the teeth and the jaw. The best are made by a dentist to ensure that they give maximum protection to your teeth. A correctly fitted mouthguard may save smashed teeth and the expense of replacement.

## Helmets

Head injuries are extremely serious. Helmets are designed to protect your skull and should be able to withstand an impact which could occur in the particular sport. Helmets should be light and comfortable and should not obstruct your vision. Helmets are essential in any sport where the head may be endangered.

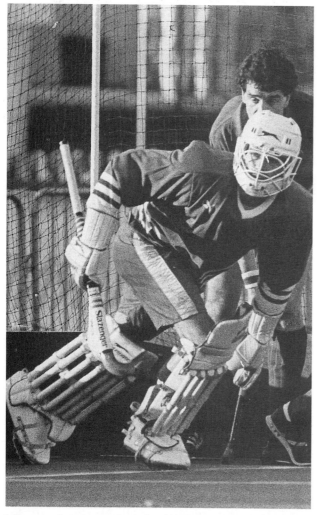

Many schools and clubs encourage young players to wear the correct gear.

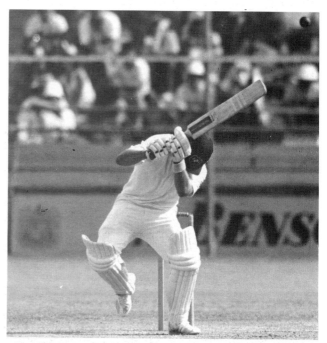

A helmet saves this batsman from possible head injury.

## Wetsuits

Wetsuits are used primarily as protection against cold. They can also protect the body against bumps and bruises. Waterskiing should never be performed without a ski safety jacket and a wetsuit, which gives protection for sensitive areas when the skier hits the water at high speed.

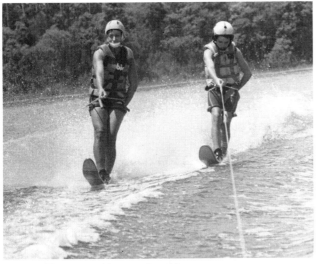

Protective gear for waterskiers.

## Padding

Padding protects bones, muscles, joints and organs. Knee pads are worn by volleyball players and shoulder pads protect the soft tissue of rugby players. Shin pads are worn by soccer and hockey players and often save painful injury to the skin.

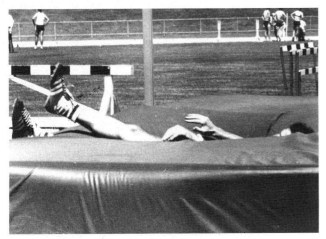

A soft landing for this high-jumper.

## Taping

Taping the ankle is considered a necessity by some footballers and players of sports where extreme pressure is placed on the ankle. *Taping should be done only by experts.*

## Dangerous articles

Players must not wear items that can cause injury to themselves and others. Earrings have been responsible for torn ears, rings and watches for gashes to other people, and neckchains for damage to the neck area. Long, sharp fingernails cause nasty gashes. There should be no item worn on the body or on clothing that can cause damage to yourself or to others.

# The rules of the game

The rules of the game are there to protect players, so it is in your interests to observe them. Some injuries occur because players deliberately break a rule and, in doing so, cause injury to another player. You can help stop this by supporting the decisions of umpires or referees.

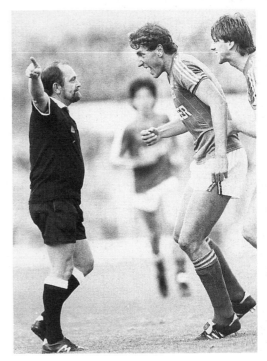

Referees and umpires should be obeyed. Their decisions help protect players from injury.

# Facilities

A safe, well-organised environment will help reduce injury. A safe environment should include:

- safety fences that are placed well back from the competition area to minimise player collision
- safe surfaces that have no potholes, and which, in the case of indoor sports, are not slippery
- outdoor playing surfaces situated across the line of the rising or setting sun so that goals or wickets are not directly in the glare
- well-maintained equipment; for example, nets should have no jutting surfaces or loose wire, posts should be smooth and padded;
- changing rooms with showers, toilets and a first-aid room
- a telephone in the rooms or nearby for immediate summoning of expert help in the case of injury.

# Injuries in sport

This next section is intended to give you a basic insight into action first-aid people usually take when a player is injured. It is *not* intended to make you an expert in treating injuries, and *on no account should you attempt to treat an injury yourself* without proper medical advice.

There are two main types of injury in sport.

- *Soft tissue injuries* are injuries to any tissue except bones. They account for over 90 per cent of sports injuries and fall into two groups:
  - open wounds where there is external bleeding
  - closed wounds such as sprains, strains and tears, where blood escapes from the circulatory system into body tissue.
- *Hard tissue injuries* are injuries to the bones of the body.

# Procedure in the case of an injury

If an injury occurs in competition or training, officials normally:

- *stop* the game or training session, quickly note the time of the accident and go to the injured player.
- *look* for any change in colour, size or shape of the area injured. If a limb has been injured, it can be compared with the uninjured one. Obvious changes in shape indicate a possible fracture or dislocation.
- *feel* gently for any swelling or tenderness around the injured part. They never prod or jab as this can cause further injury. If a limb can be touched in this way without intense pain, the injury is usually not a fracture. However, in children under 12, their ligaments are stronger than their bones, so a bone is more likely to break than a ligament is to tear. Officials therefore treat swelling and bruising around a child's joints as a possible fracture. Movement should never be forced to see if a leg or arm has been badly injured. Any movement should be attempted only by the injured player and only if the player feels comfortable doing so and without being rushed.
- *apply* first-aid procedures for open or closed wounds of soft tissue.
- *call* for medical assistance if a fracture is suspected. As medical assistance is normally easily available, the victim should not be moved.

## Open wounds

With open wounds, treatment will depend on the extent of the wound. Control of bleeding is always most important. If the wound is minor, it is normally cleansed and dressed. If the wound is extensive or has foreign bodies in it, a doctor must treat it. Doctors often give tetanus shots for open wounds.

In the case of burns, cool or iced water is run gently over the burn, and air should be kept from the area. This can be achieved by dribbling water over a bandage placed over the burn. All burns which break the skin should be inspected by a doctor to prevent infection. Blisters, whether from burns or any other cause, should not be broken as this increases the likelihood of infection and extends healing time.

## Closed wounds

Treatment for closed wounds where a fracture is not suspected is normally based on the I.C.E. formula. I.C.E. stands for:
- Ice
- Compression
- Elevation.

### Ice

Doctors believe that ice packs applied immediately to an injury can have a number of desirable effects:
- swelling and inflammation are reduced
- bleeding in the tissues of the injured area is reduced
- muscle spasm is reduced
- numbness and reduction of pain are achieved.

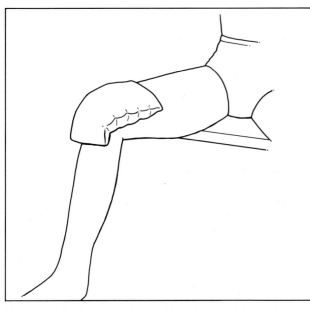

**Figure 5.1:** Application of ice to an injured knee.

The ice treatment should continue for periods of 20 minutes on and 20 minutes off for the first few hours. Applications of ice can be continued over the next two days. Ice should never touch the skin; it should always be applied as an ice pack. An ice pack can be made by wrapping ice in a wet towel. Stored packs can be prepared by freezing water in styrofoam cups. The top few centimetres of the cup can be stripped off and the exposed ice can be used to massage the injured area over a wet cloth.

### Compression

Ice treatment is accompanied by compression of the injured area with a crêpe bandage which helps to limit swelling. However, the bandage should not be so tight that it causes pain or prevents the normal blood circulation. Officials watch for danger signs such as a bluish colour of the skin around the edges of the bandage or a numbing tingle, both of which indicate that the bandage is too tight.

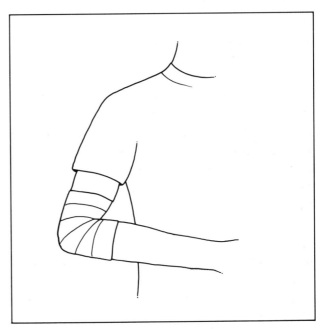

**Figure 5.2:** Compression applied to an injured elbow.

### Elevation

If movement does not cause pain, the injured area is elevated above the level of the heart. This helps reduce the amount of blood flowing to the injured area and helps drain waste products from the injury.

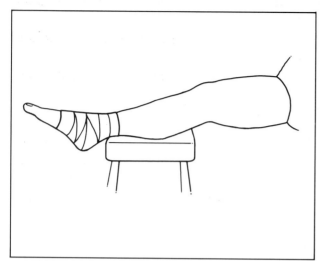

**Figure 5.3:** Elevation of an injured ankle.

Remember, these procedures are applied to minor injuries. Emergency treatment to head or spinal injuries except to save life should not be attempted and medical help should be sought immediately.

# Soft tissue injuries

The most common soft tissue injuries in sport involve:

- skin
- muscles
- tendons
- ligaments
- cartilage.

## Skin

Skin injuries are very common. Most are minor and respond to basic first aid.

### Grazing

*Description:* In grazing, only the surface of the skin is broken.
*Cause:* Collision with hard surfaces especially the ground.
*Prevention:*
- Well-grassed playing surfaces.
- Protective clothing.

*Treatment:* Clean with water, dry and apply antiseptic ointment if available; leave uncovered if possible.

## Deep cuts

*Description:* Deep opening in the skin, exposing underlying tissue.
*Cause:* Collision with a sharp object.
*Prevention:*
- Well-kept equipment; no jagged edges.
- Fields well kept and often inspected.
- Removal of sharp objects from clothing and the body, and cutting or taping of long fingernails.

*Treatment:* Stop bleeding by pressing with a clean cloth. Use water to clean out dirt, grit etc. Dab on antiseptic. If shallow, cover with gauze and adhesive tape; if deep, seek medical advice.

## Punctures

*Description:* Deep wound with small opening in skin.
*Cause:* Punctured by sharp object such as a spike or javelin.
*Prevention:*
- Well-kept equipment; no jagged edges.
- Care when using throwing objects.

*Treatment:* Seek medical advice.

## Burns

*Description:* Damage to one, two or all three layers of skin.
*Cause:* Friction during a slide or from a rope; exposure to sun.
*Prevention:*
- Care in performing rope exercises.
- Protective clothing.
- Wearing sunscreen and hats.

*Treatment:* Treat as for a graze. Clean with running water, dry; leave uncovered if possible.

## Blistering

*Description:* A raised section of skin with fluid between the layers.
*Causes:* Friction; rowers and gymnasts

returning to training after a long lay-off may get blistered hands; athletes may get blistered feet from poorly fitting shoes.

*Prevention:*
- Gradual toughening of the skin before hard training.
- Good shoes and socks.

*Treatment:* Clean with antiseptic. If the blister fluid is released leave skin in place, cover with a gauze pad, then adhesive tape.

## Chafing

*Description:* Irritation and minor skin damage.
*Causes:* Tight clothing; rough seams; continual rubbing of skin on skin.
*Prevention:*
- Suitable clothing.
- Vaseline applications in areas such as between the legs and under the arms.

## Bruising

*Description:* Swelling and discoloration which indicates bleeding into the soft tissues under the skin.
*Causes:* A hard knock, colliding with another player or object; falls, especially on a hard surface.

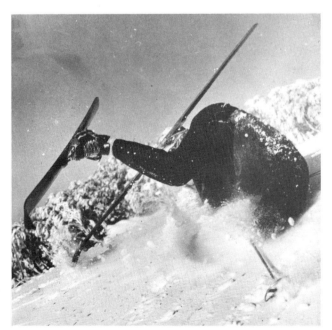

Bruising can result from a heavy fall.

*Prevention:*
- Protective clothing.
- Padded field equipment such as goal posts.
- Skill in using equipment such as hockey sticks.

*Treatment:* Use I.C.E. to restrict the swelling.

# Muscles

Muscle injuries are common in all body-contact sports and sports that involve fast, sudden and vigorous movements. The damage can range from a slight strain to a painful tear.

### Muscle strain

*Description:* Some muscle fibres are strained leading to pain and tenderness. The area does not discolour as there is little bleeding.
*Cause:* Muscle strain can occur through even such simple movements as picking up a bat when muscles are "cold".
*Prevention:* Warm-up and stretching exercises.
*Treatment:* Rest injured part. Apply I.C.E. treatment.

### Muscular tears

*Description:* Muscular tears or pulled muscles, as they are commonly called, are more serious than strains. Many fibres in the muscle tear and bruising occurs, which indicates bleeding. It may take several days for bruising to appear in a very deep tear.
*Causes:* Muscle tears are common in fast, vigorous sports. Track and field athletes and footballers often tear hamstrings, wicket-keepers the groin muscle, and netballers their calf muscles. Tears are common in other fast-moving sports such as squash, fencing, hockey, tennis and surfing. These tears result from too much strain on a muscle caused by:
- inadequate warm-up or the player's muscles have cooled down between games
- lack of flexibility caused by inadequate daily stretching exercises

- fatigue near the end of a game when the player has less control over muscle action
- poor training methods where the workload was increased too fast.

*Prevention:*
- Proper warming-up exercises.
- Well-designed training programme.

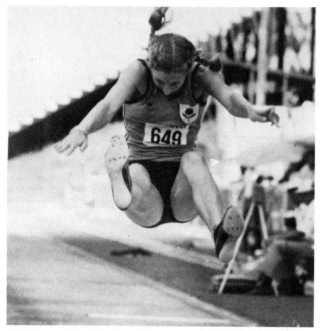

Proper warming up and stretching exercises prevent muscle tears when competing.

To prevent the injury worsening, it is important that players stop immediately they feel a sharp pain, a pulling, a knotting or tightness in the muscle, and apply I.C.E. to the area.

## Cramp

*Description:* A sudden and sustained contraction of a muscle that can last for a few minutes or several hours. In a few rare cases, muscle cramp can be so severe it can cause broken bones.
*Causes:* Poor training and preparation, and lack of fitness; an unbalanced diet lacking in essential minerals, particularly calcium.
*Prevention:*
- Well-designed training programme.
- High level of fitness.
- Fresh fruit, vegetables and cereals in the diet.

*Treatment:* Stretch muscle and massage firmly.

## Stitch

*Description:* A sharp, sudden pain across the top part of the abdomen which sometimes stretches up into the side of the body. It is a type of muscle cramp. Some doctors feel it is the diaphragm that is cramping.
*Causes:* Eating before exercise; lack of fitness in the early days of a training programme.
*Prevention:*
- Not eating before exercise.
- High level of fitness.

*Treatment:* Push fingers into the area that hurts and bend over, exhaling forcibly.

## Tendons

Tendons attach muscles to the bone. During movement, the muscle contracts and lengthens but the tendons do not. In areas such as the wrists and sides of the ankles the tendons are covered by a "synovial" sheath which produces a lubricant called synovial fluid. Most damage to tendons is due to internal stress rather than to external violence. During exercise, tension and friction on the tendons increase.

### Tendonitis

*Description:* Tendonitis is a common tendon injury. Tendonitis is inflammation and swelling of the tendon. The tendon is most sore in the morning when you first get out of bed. As you move about and warm up, the tenderness disappears. However, the injury remains.

Tendonitis is common in the achilles tendon of long-distance runners, in the elbow of tennis players and in the shoulder of swimmers. Recent studies have revealed tendonitis in swimmers as young as 15.
*Cause:* A long period of repetitive stress during which tight muscles pull on the tendons.
*Prevention:* Stretching exercises.

*Note:* The tenderness felt in the morning is a warning sign to seek medical help. If you ignore it and warm up until the tenderness disappears, you will probably cause serious problems which may appear later in life.

# Tenosynovitis

*Description:* Tenosynovitis is irritation and inflammation of the synovial sheath.
*Cause:* Repetitive use of the joint muscles and tendons.
*Prevention:*
- Adequate warm-up and stretching.
- Correct technique.

## Complete rupture

*Description:* Tendon rupture is:
- the tendon separating from the bone
- the tendon separating from the muscle
- the tendon tearing apart.

It is a serious injury. A tendon rupture can end a sporting career or, at the least, put the player out for a long time. A ruptured tendon will "pop" when it breaks and the player will be in instant agony. Medical assistance must be sought immediately and I.C.E. applied while waiting. The most common tendon that ruptures is the achilles tendon in the heel.
*Causes:* Tight, inflexible muscles which place a greater strain on tendons; sudden vigorous activity when muscles are tight and cold.
*Prevention:*
- A well-designed training programme.
- Warm-up exercises, especially stretching exercises.

# Ligaments

Ligaments attach one bone to another in a joint, giving joint stability within its normal range of movement.

## Sprained ligaments

*Description:* This occurs when some of the ligament fibres are overstretched. These account for about 98 per cent of ligament injuries.
*Causes:* Sprained ligaments are most common in fast, vigorous sports such as football, hockey and basketball, where players can land awkwardly or suffer external violence.

*Prevention:*
- Strength, flexibility and balance exercises.
- High level of skill in the sport.

## Torn or ruptured ligaments

*Description:* This occurs when ligaments are completely torn or even wrenched from the bone.
*Cause:* External violence.
*Prevention:*
- Strength, flexibility and balance exercises.
- High level of skill in the sport.

All ligament damage should be treated by a doctor to prevent worsening of the injury. Although some torn or ruptured ligaments may re-attach themselves to the bone, others require expert surgery.

# Cartilage

Cartilage is found in different forms in the body. It contains no blood vessels and does not repair easily. In sports injuries two types of cartilage that are most commonly damaged are:
- articular cartilage which is attached to the bone surfaces in a joint and allows smooth movement between bones
- wedge-shaped pieces of cartilage, which are found in mobile joints such as the knee and help the bones fit more snugly together. Each piece of wedge-shaped cartilage is called a meniscus.

## Articular damage

*Description:* Damage to articular cartilage occurs in the more mobile joints of the body – the elbow, hip, ankle, and especially the knee. The cartilage can become rough and might then require surgical repair.
*Causes:* Overuse of the joint; malalignment of the joint, causing excessive pressure on a small area.
*Prevention:*
- High level of fitness and skill.
- Warming up before an activity.
- Avoiding overload on joints by strengthening the supporting muscles.

## Meniscal tears

*Description:* Meniscal tears occur most commonly in the knee joint and require surgical repair.

*Causes:* Violent knock; violent wrenching or turning.

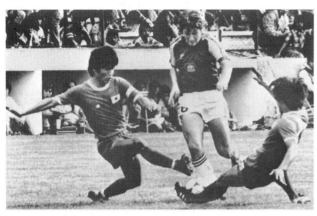

Tackles can cause damage to the mobile joints of the body.

*Prevention:*
- High level of fitness, skill and balance.
- Warming up before an activity.
- Care in movement.
- Avoiding overload on joints by strengthening the supporting muscles.

# Hard tissue injuries

Hard tissue injuries are, fortunately, not as common as injuries to soft tissues. They occur mostly in body-contact sports, although skiers, horseriders and gymnasts can break bones if they have a fall. A broken bone is called a fracture, and the two types of fracture are the complete fracture and the stress fracture. Players with suspected fractures should not be moved except by medical personnel.

## Complete fracture

A complete fracture is when the bone is broken into two pieces. The injury causes extreme pain especially if the player is moved.

A broken bone must not be moved, because the broken edge may:
- cut a nerve, leaving the person paralysed, especially in a spinal injury
- puncture a lung in the case of a broken rib
- cut a blood vessel
- puncture the skin leaving the injury open to infection.

Only doctors can set fractures.

## Stress fracture

A stress fracture occurs when cracks appear in the surface of the bone. Stress fractures are most common in the hand, shin and bones of the feet.

In sport, stress fractures are often caused by running long distances on hard ground. Medical assistance must be sought for a suspected stress fracture.

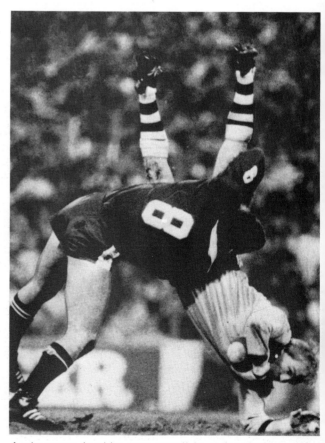

A vigorous tackle can result in a fracture.

# Joint injuries

Joints are the meeting place of bones. They are also the place where you find soft tissues such as muscles, ligaments and cartilage. Damage at the joints can occur to either soft or hard tissue or both and is usually painful.

People who play sports that involve fast, violent turns and rotation, especially if it is a body-contact sport, are most likely to injure their joints. Damage to a joint can range from a minor sprain to a complete dislocation. The two most mobile joints, the knee and shoulder, are the most unstable and are very prone to joint damage.

## Knee joint injuries

You can see from figure 5.4 that the knee is a complex joint.

Injury to a knee joint can be not only very painful but also long lasting. Special care should be taken to avoid such injuries.

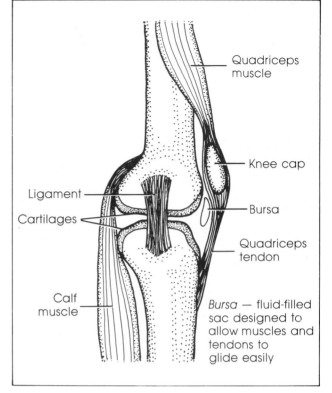

**Figure 5.4:** Places where the knee can be injured.

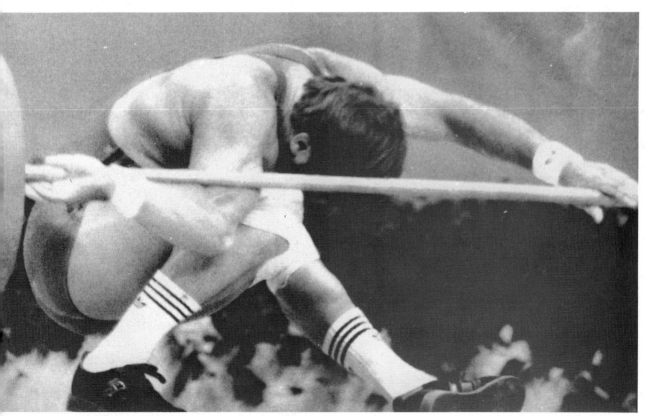

The falling bar hit this weightlifter in the head and caused him to dislocate his right elbow and strain his right knee.

*Description:* Damage to the knee can be done to any or all of the following:

- the cartilage
- the knee cap tendons
- the ligaments
- the muscles
- the knee cap
- the bursae.

A sign of damage is continued pain, swelling or "locking" of the joint.

*Causes:* Violent wrenching or twisting of the knee, excessive jumping particularly on hard surfaces. It is a common injury in basketball, netball, volleyball and football.

*Prevention:*

- Care in movement.
- High level of skill.
- Exercises to strengthen muscles surrounding the knee and to improve balance.
- Cushioned footwear.

Continual pain around the knee is a sign that treatment should be sought.

## Elbow joint injuries

The elbow joint depends for stability on tendons and muscles. Its ligaments are fairly weak.

*Description:* The most common injuries are to the tendons that support the joint. People often talk about "tennis elbow", which is a form of tendonitis. Athletes playing racquet sports have to be particularly aware of this.

*Causes:* Overuse of the muscles of the forearm; incorrect throwing action; incorrect grip on racquets or bats.

*Prevention:*

- Ensure racquets and bats have the correct weight and grip for you. Ensure tennis racquets are strung at the correct tension.
- Ensure that you develop a correct throwing technique.

## Shoulder joint injuries

The shoulder joint is similar to the knee joint in that it relies heavily on soft tissues for its stability.

*Description:* Damage to the shoulder joint can range from sprains or tears in soft tissue to complete dislocation. Dislocation occurs when the head of the humerus bone is forced out of the shoulder capsule. Sometimes damage to the ligaments supporting the capsule is so extensive that the joint never regains its stability. If the bone continues to slip out of position in normal, everyday actions, surgery is necessary.

*Causes:* Abnormally shallow shoulder socket; external force from hard body contact or a fall; overuse from racquet and bat games, swimming, throwing or bowling.

*Prevention:*

- Strengthen muscle in shoulder.
- Flexibility exercises.
- Shoulder pads.

## Ankle joint injuries

*Description:* Injuries to the ankle range from a ligament strain to a fracture of a bone. Sprained ligaments greatly reduce the ability of the ankle joint to perform its many functions.

*Causes:* Sprained or broken ankles are common among players whose sport involves running, twisting, turning or jumping.

*Prevention:*

- Flexibility, strengthening and balance exercises.
- High level of skill.
- Well-designed footwear.

If an ankle is damaged, it may require an X-ray to determine whether the injury is a sprain or a fracture. A permanently weak ankle will result if a player does not treat a sprain correctly the first time. Proper treatment, support, and corrective exercises are necessary if the ankle is to regain its former stability.

# Other common injuries

## Winding

Players can get "winded" by a blow to the pit of the stomach which, for a short time, stops the action of the diaphragm and takes away the breath. When winding occurs, the player is placed on his or her back with legs bent and feet on the ground. The player should then take deep breaths. On no account should the legs be pumped towards the chest or the chest thumped, in case other injuries have occurred.

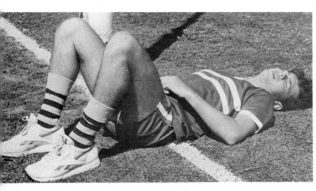

A winded player should lie down with legs bent and take deep breaths.

## Heat exhaustion

Heat exhaustion is caused when a player becomes so overheated that water loss becomes critical. Heat exhaustion affects the body gradually. Tiredness and weakness are the early signs and, as the body dehydrates, the player becomes exhausted. If enough fluid is lost, the blood volume decreases to the stage where the player goes into shock.

Athletes performing in marathons, long-distance bike-riding and triathlons can lose about 4 litres of fluid in an hour. These athletes must have regular intakes of cool water while performing. If athletes suffer from heat exhaustion, they are:

- placed in shade and clothing loosened
- cooled down with water
- given fluids.

Medical assistance should be sought.

## Nose bleed

A common injury in many sports is nose bleed. The normal treatment is to:

- sit the player down with head forward
- get the player to pinch the nostrils together for several minutes
- apply an ice pack to the back of the neck and forehead.

## Ear injury

Bleeding from the ear after a blow to the head can indicate a serious injury, so medical assistance must be sought immediately. The ears should never be blocked to stop bleeding. Normally, the player lies down and, while waiting for medical assistance, officials keep a careful check on consciousness, airways, breathing and circulation.

## Eye injury

Any injury to the eye should be treated only by a doctor. The injured eye can be covered with a pad as this usually gives some relief while the player is taken to the doctor.

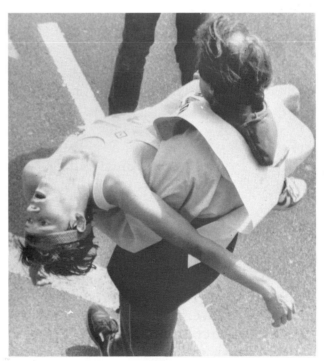

A heat exhaustion victim.

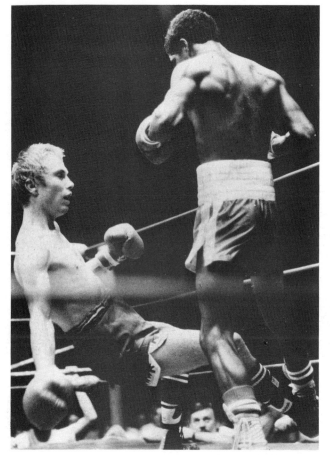

A blow to the head in boxing can result in injuries ranging from a nose bleed to ear or eye problems, or worse.

## Abdomen injury

If a player has suffered a blow to the abdomen and appears to be more than winded, immediate medical assistance must be called as internal organs may have been damaged. Only a doctor will be able to determine the extent of abdominal injury. The player's legs are *never* pumped.

## Chest injury

Chest injuries are common in contact sports and can be dangerous, as a broken rib can puncture the spleen or a lung. If the player complains of shortness of breath, difficulty in taking a deep breath, or cannot move without causing pain, the injury is treated as a possible fracture.

Under no circumstances should the chest be strapped by non-medical personnel.

## Shin splints

Shin splints refers to a pain that runs up the shins. It is common in long-distance runners and is caused by the muscles of the front of the leg pulling slightly away from the bone, resulting in pain and inflammation. It is an injury resulting from overuse.

If you suffer from shin splints:
- ensure you have good footwear
- perform lower leg stretching exercises
- avoid training on hard surfaces.

## Injury to the teeth

Teeth can be damaged in many sports. If teeth are knocked out, they should be collected and washed. Expert dental assistance should be sought immediately.

## Fractured collar bone

A fractured collar bone is the most common of all fractures. It is usually caused by a fall or a very hard collision. Support the arm in a sling and seek medical treatment.

During the growth-spurt stage of adolescence, some areas of immature bone development are subject to extra stress during sport. The most commonly affected areas are the foot arch, the heel, the area just below the kneecap, the hip and the mid and lower spine. In the past, pains in these regions were regarded as "growing pains"; however, the area can become "arthritic" in later years owing to inadequate treatment. Therefore, recurrent pain after sport should be evaluated by a professional who specialises in sports medicine.

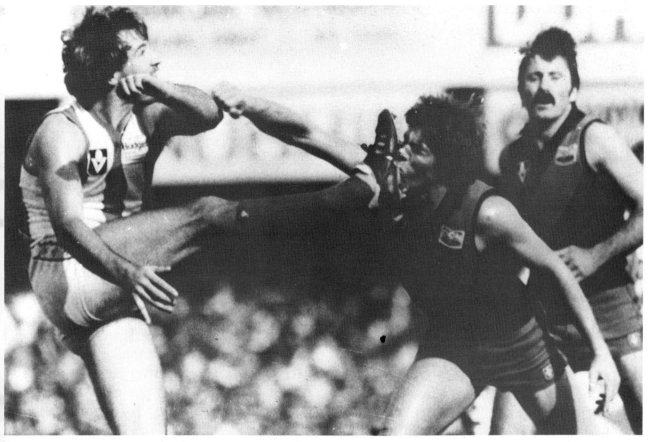

The possibility of teeth injuries in Australian football are obvious here, where a player is kicked in the face while trying to smother the ball.

## Dislocated finger or thumb

This type of injury is common in ball sports such as football, cricket and softball. Apply I.C.E., and seek prompt professional treatment.

## "Cork" or haematoma

This is internal bleeding and bruising of a muscle often caused by a heavy collision in body-contact sports. The area usually undergoes a fibrous change resulting in shortening of the muscle length. Therefore, early treatment and subsequent stretching exercises are most important.

# Rehabilitation

Rehabilitation is the process of restoring both the injured part and the rest of the body to the level of fitness and skill present before injury.

To aid in rehabilitation, it is important that athletes exercise the uninjured parts of the body as much as possible while their injury is healing. Exercises should be those recommended by the doctor. Every day away from training will require two days of training to restore the athlete to the level of fitness achieved before the injury. And remember, you should not compete until rehabilitation is complete.

# 6

# Sport, society and you

## Development of sport

Throughout history, most people had to work very long hours to provide themselves with food and shelter to survive. This meant that they did not have the leisure time to play organised sport. Sport belonged to the wealthy who had both the money and the time to enjoy leisure activities. However, during the eighteenth and nineteenth centuries, increasing industrialisation drew many people from the country areas to the cities to find work in factories and offices. Over a long period of time, these people gained shorter working hours, which allowed more time for leisure. To fill their spare time, people turned to many things – education, reading, entertainment and sport.

## Sport in Britain

At this time the foundations of modern sport were established. Many of Britain's sports, for example, rugby and football, have greatly influenced the development of sport throughout the world.

Many factors contributed to how sport developed in Britain and these stemmed from the traditions of the school system. In the nineteenth century "organised games" became a feature of all private schools and were seen as a means of character training and providing self-discipline for later life. The elementary schools, which were for the majority of children, offered exercises and drill. This was partly due to a lack of space but also provided a means of controlling large number of pupils by discipline.

One of the major developments in state schools at the beginning of the century was the introduction of gymnastics, which had been imported from Sweden and gradually replaced ten drill type exercises.

The differing traditions of sport seen in the private and state sectors of education have continued until recent times.

Within this century the increase of leisure has led to more people being able to take part in sport. Public sports facilities have developed, giving individuals far greater access to a wide variety of activities.

Britain in this age is a nation extremely interested in sport. Whether as participants or spectators sport can both unite and divide us as a people, as we play or discuss sporting events together.

There are numerous examples of sporting events that create enthusiasm throughout the country such as the F.A. Cup Final, the Oxford and Cambridge boat race, the Grand National and Wimbledon tennis.

However, in spite of their interest in sport only a small proportion of British people play sport regularly. By 1993 the Sports Council aims to have 5 million more men and women participating in sport.

Love of sport is also an important part of life in other countries. More than one-quarter of the world's population watched the Olympic Games on television.

Because sport has such an important role in the modern world, some people have begun to study sport and its place in society. People who study society are called sociologists. Sociologists explain patterns of behaviour in society using scientific methods. When sociologists focus on sport, we call their study the *sociology of sport*.

# The sociology of sport

In the sociology of sport we look at:
● the behaviour patterns of players, officials, spectators and sponsors
● cultural influences on sport
● sport's role in society
● institutions and organisations dealing with sport.

Sometimes sociologists turn to psychologists to aid them in their studies. Psychologists study the physical and mental development of people and can help in skill and personality development in sport.

When we examine sport and society, we must first define what "sport" means.

## What is sport?

The word "sport" is used so often that we are surprised to find that it is not an easy word to define. After all, we know that cricket, netball, hockey and football are sports. However, are camping, hunting and windsurfing sports? Is touch football a sport? When a primary school student plays continuous cricket, is it a sport? One method of solving the difficulty of defining sport is to distinguish between play, recreation, games and sport. However, remember that we are considering only active physical activities. Games such as cards and chess are not considered in this study.

### Play

Play is physical activity in which there are:
● no formal rules
● no pressure
● no winners or losers
● no set time
● no defined playing area.

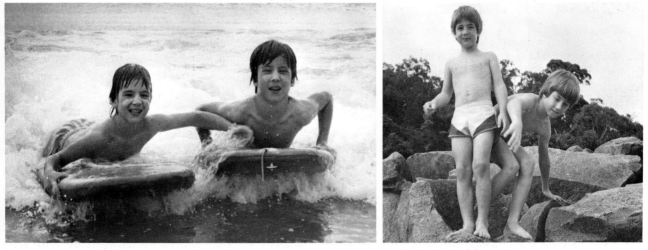

Play is informal physical activity with no formal rules and no winners and losers.

Thus, in play, people enjoy spontaneous physical activity. If you go swimming with a group of friends, or kick a ball around in a park, then you are at play. You are involved in physical activity just for fun.

## Recreation

Recreation is more planned than play but also has:
● no winners or losers
● no highly organised rules.
Examples of recreation are non-competitive fishing, walking, surfing and skiing.

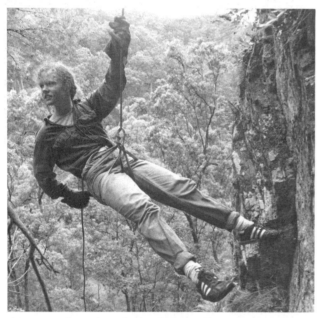

A recreational activity demanding a high level of skill.

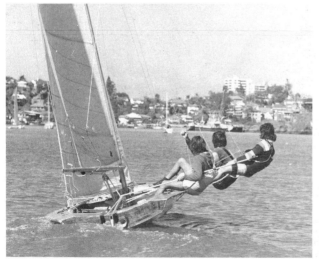

Yachting can be recreation or a sport.

## Games

Games are more organised than recreation and play. They involve:
● an agreed playing area
● an agreed time limit
● a higher level of skill than is needed for play
● rules which can change
● contest between two people or between two groups, where one person or group is the winner.

Thus, if ten players play five-a-side hockey using some of the rules of traditional hockey and at the same time keep score, then they are playing a *game*; if students at primary school play continuous cricket with rules adapted by their teacher to suit their age group, they are playing a *game*. Games, therefore, are more formal than *play* but less structured than *sport*.

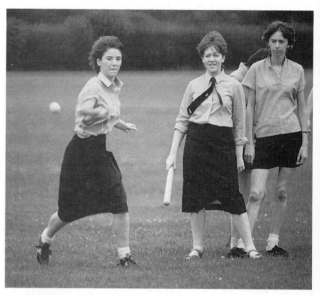

Rounders is very popular among both men and women.

## Sport

Sport is much more organised than play, recreation or games. Sport involves:
● set rules, area and time
● set positions for team players
● usually vigorous physical activity
● complex physical skills which are applied throughout the set time

- serious training and preparation
- competition between individuals or teams where winning is very important
- satisfaction for players coming not only from the enjoyment of playing the sport but also from winning awards, prizes and even applause from supporters.

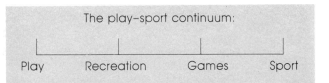

The play–sport continuum:

| | | | |
|---|---|---|---|
| Play | Recreation | Games | Sport |

As physical activity moves from play to sport, the following occur:
- the physical activity becomes less spontaneous and more controlled by rules
- individuals put in more effort and time in learning skills, preparing tactics and playing to win
- spectators become more evident and involved
- the rewards involve personal enjoyment but more and more also include gaining awards, prizes and/or recognition.

(Adapted from ideas of Harry Edwards, *Sociology of Sport*, Illinois: Dorsey Press, 1983.)

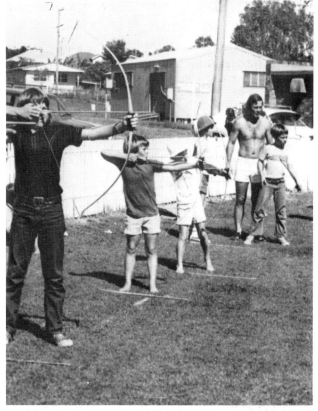

Archery, a recreation or a sport enjoyed in safety by people of all ages.

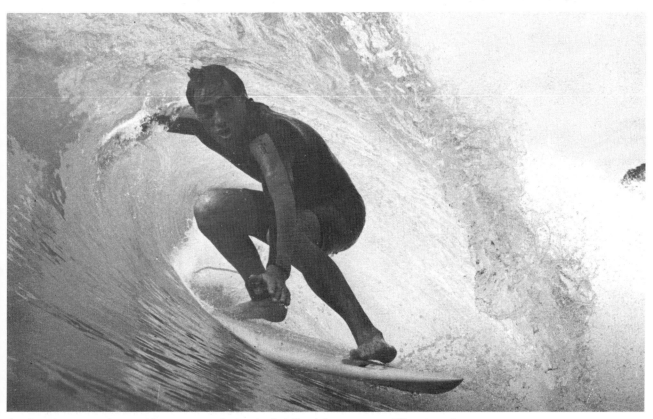

Surfing is a sport requiring a great deal of skill at the competitive level.

# People and sport

When we examine sport, we find there are five main groups of people involved:

- the players
- the officials
- the spectators
- the media
- the sponsors.

## The players

Sociologists have found that different people have different reasons for playing sport. These reasons include:

- *Enjoyment.* Many players play simply because they enjoy themselves.

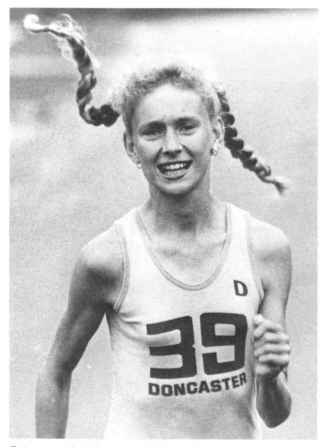

Enjoyment: the fun of being fit.

- *Socializing.* Many players join sporting clubs to mix with others who enjoy similar activities. Mixing is not restricted to the playing fields. Players become involved in support programmes such as fund-raising, and often develop a network of friends based on sporting contacts. Sometimes the friendships are more important than winning or losing or even playing the sport.

- *Health.* Many people play sport to keep their bodies fit and healthy.

- *Release.* Many players find that vigorous sporting activity helps rid them of the tensions of everyday life. Aggression can be used to advantage and without harm on the sports field.

- *Competition.* Some players have a strong competitive nature. They like to test themselves in a win-lose situation. Sport provides an outlet for this.

- *Excitement.* Some players find that sport provides them with an excitement they cannot find in their everyday routine. Sport can also give them a taste of danger as they push their bodies to greater feats.

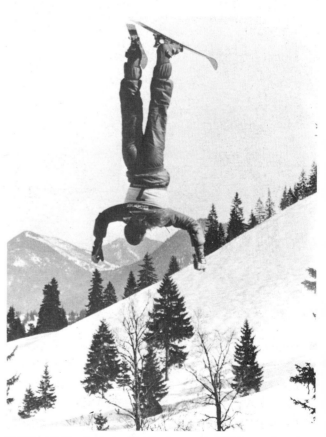

Thrills of "hot dogging", a most dangerous activity.

- *Self-expression.* Some players find that sport is an area where they can express themselves in movement.
- *Self-testing.* Some players with high levels of skill wish to test their bodies even further. They are even prepared to suffer pain as they push their performance level higher.
- *Self-esteem.* Some people who have natural physical talents train themselves to perform brilliantly, thus developing esteem for themselves through success in the sporting field.
- *Aesthetic awareness:* Some players admire the grace and beauty of their chosen sport and are prepared to train hard to develop the skill to provide beauty for themselves and spectators.

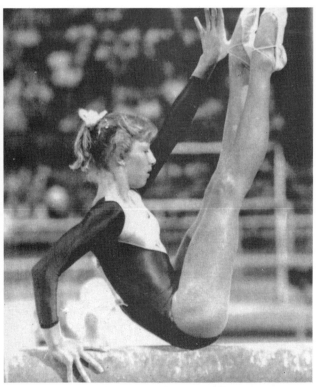

The grace and form of gymnastics.

- *Career opportunities.* Some players have special talents which can lead them into professional sports where they can combine love of sport with earning a living.
- *Encouragement.* Many young players enter sports through parental, peer or school encouragement.

## Player involvement

Whatever reasons people have for participating in sport, they have to be able to:
- train to develop the skills of the sport
- learn the rules
- spend time working on tactics.

Players also have to learn to accept advice or instruction from coach and captain. In team sports, players must learn to work as members of a team rather than as individuals. Players also have to learn how to behave based on an acceptable code.

## Players and ethics

A code of ethics is an organised set of ideas about the way to behave based on the belief that certain things are "right" and other things are "wrong". Ethics can vary, however, as people's beliefs about right and wrong vary.

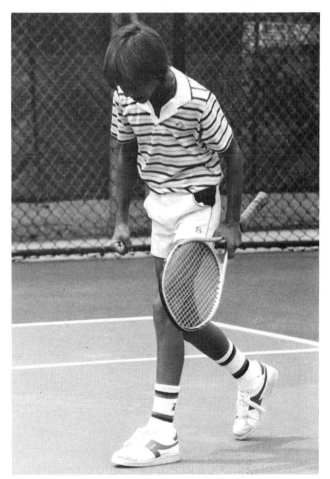

Sometimes it is difficult not to show frustration.

Traditionally most players shared common ethics in sport, which included beliefs that players:

- played sport to the best of their ability; this was more important than winning or losing
- treated team mates and opponents with respect, avoiding harmful tactics
- never cheated or tried to win by unfair methods
- behaved with dignity
- never bragged about winning or moaned about defeat; they never blamed defeat on others
- accepted the umpire's/referee's decision without question, even when they felt the decision was wrong.

Today, not everyone agrees on these sporting ethics. For many, the main aim is to win rather than to "play the game". Some players are prepared to create scenes to shake the confidence of opponents so that they will make mistakes. Some professionals believe that, with so much money at stake, they must question controversial decisions made by umpires or referees.

## Players as heroes

The tradition of the player as a hero is a long one dating back to ancient Greece. However, through the mass media today, players become heroes to millions. Reasons for this include:

- *Media coverage.* As the media continually provide information about sporting stars, they become everyday topics of conversation.
- *Appreciation of excellence.* Many fans admire the tremendously high level of performance of a sports star.
- *National pride.* Players who succeed in international competition often become national heroes.
- *Glamour.* Many fans follow sporting careers to share in what they see as their hero's "glamorous" life – fame, money, travel and excitement. Often fans are not aware of the hard work, the long hours of

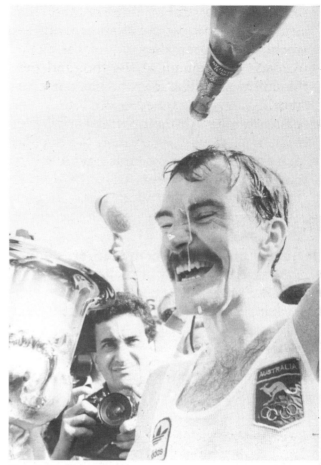

The thrill of victory.

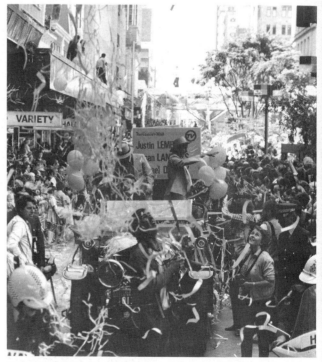

Sporting stars are given a hero's welcome when they return home.

practice, the loneliness of the hotel rooms as players follow competitions around the world, the injuries, the continual struggle to reach and remain at the top, and the difficulty of adjusting to life once a sporting career is ended.

- *Affection.* As cameras zero in on individuals striving to do their best, spectators come to feel they know and like the player.

# The officials

There are three groups of officials:
- coaches
- umpires, referees, line umpires
- organisers.

## Coaches

Coaches are responsible for the skills, tactics and ethics of their players. They:

- encourage players to enjoy their sport
- encourage ethical behaviour, such as respect for all players and referees or umpires
- balance the desire to win with the need to play the game in the correct spirit
- are aware of the needs and abilities of players and try to protect them from injury.

## Umpires, referees, line umpires

Traditionally, the job of these people was to control the game according to the rules. Most were volunteers who gave up their time for love of the sport.

Referees and umpires are experts on the rules of their game and have to pass a series of practical and theoretical examinations before they can officiate at a top-level game. In many sports they must maintain a high level of fitness.

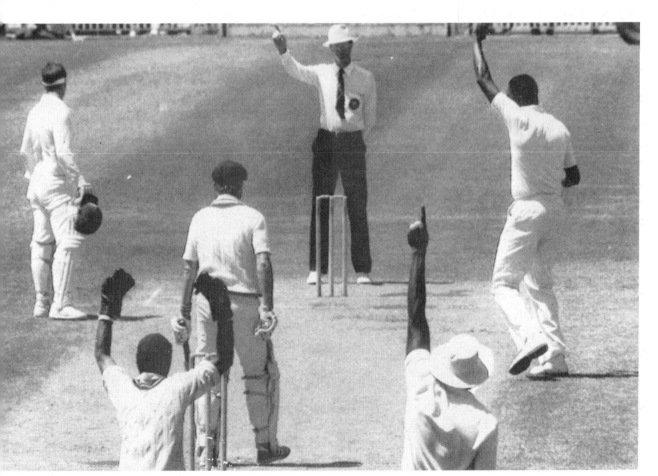

Accepting the umpire's decision.

Their job has grown more difficult today. More players are prepared to question decisions aggressively, a factor which often causes conflict. Secondly, important sporting contests are almost always televised. Controversial decisions are subject to the scrutiny of armchair spectators and sports commentators who can see the play from many different camera angles through slow-motion replays. Sporting authorities increasingly have brought in a system of fines and penalties for players in an attempt to end player abuse of umpires and to "clean up" player behaviour. Umpires know that they must be clear about rules because of the importance of the contest to the players.

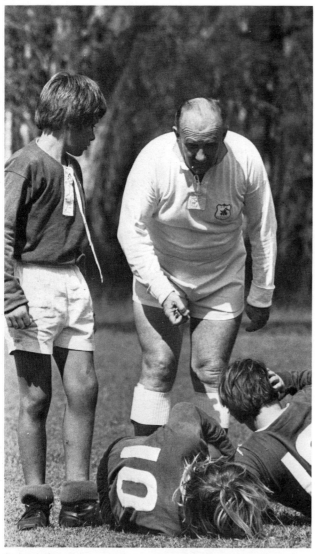

The referee is concerned with the safety of players as well as the rules of the game.

## Organisers

Sport needs organisation. Rules are usually standardised by international bodies, national bodies oversee the sport at national level, state bodies at state level. The strength of sport lies in local branches, for it is at this level that young players first come in contact with the sport. In clubs, interested people set up facilities and organise competition. Sport is funded both by local fund-raising and government subsidies. Clubs are usually organised by a committee (see table 6.1).

**Table 6.1**

| Position | Task |
|----------|------|
| Chair | overall responsibility for the club |
| Secretary | controls records and handles correspondence |
| Treasurer | responsible for recording finances |
| Manager | manages the team in competition |

These organisers ensure the smooth running of the club.

As sport has developed an important role in the community, sports specialists also provide information for sporting groups. University lecturers and researchers, and teacher training institutions all add to the store of knowledge available to organisers.

# Spectators

Spectators have a very important role in sport. They:
- provide funds directly through gate money when they attend matches
- provide an audience for radio and TV
- provide enthusiasm and encouragement which keep the sport going.

## What makes people spectators?

Spectators fall into four main groups:
- *Enthusiasts.* These spectators simply enjoy watching their favourite sport.
- *Mixers.* These people become spectators so that they can go to sporting outings and

share common experiences and conversation with friends.

- *Fans.* These spectators become fans of particular local, regional or national teams. The loyalty they develop to their team gives them identification with a group, and they gain pride and satisfaction when their team performs well. Their attachment to their team provides interest in their lives. Fans often travel long distances to watch their team, sometimes overseas. Defeat often causes intense disappointment, although usually the fan remains loyal to the team.
- *Parents.* Parents are among the most devoted spectators, encouraging their children to perform as well as possible.

## The role of spectators

Spectators have a role to play in sport. They can make the game better by cheering their side on, by applauding skill and sportsmanship whichever side displays it, and by showing respect for the umpires/referees. Spectators can increase their own enjoyment by understanding the finer points of rules, skills and performances.

Spectators can show their disapproval of foul play or poor behaviour. However, they can spoil sport if they become so biased that they question all decisions made against their team. They can lessen their own dignity and lower the tone of the sport by booing players or by deliberately making a noise which puts off the opposition.

Parents have a special role as spectators. They can increase the enjoyment of their children by encouraging them to play for fun and to develop skills and technique, and to abide by the ethics of the game. However, most parents are careful not to put too much pressure on children. Too much pressure can lead to children opting out because they feel that they cannot meet their parents' expectations, and so they lose their enjoyment of the sport.

This Australian newspaper article (figure 6.1) reports one of the most worrying aspects of

## Spectator violence

# PC Peta lashes cricket drunks

**SYDNEY: Constable Peta Blood, one of the casualties of last night's SCG violence, today lashed out at cricket drunks.**

She also hit out at the lack of security which allowed them to take alcohol into the ground.

Constable Blood, 21, has a badly sprained hand, cuts and bruises.

She struggled to arrest one of the brawlers.

"He had a whole bottle of scotch beside him," she said.

Constable Blood said many of the crowd of 36 000 at the ground were "pretty well inebriated".

"Something has to be done about it," she said. "It's dangerous for innocent people who want to enjoy the game."

Constable Blood and her partner were sent to The Hill to move two fans who had climbed scaffolding.

"The first one came down peacefully, but when my partner went back up the other man kicked him in the face and started punching him," she said.

"This man kicked and punched me and we both fell backwards down the stairs."

A man, 29, was remanded on bail until February 5 when he appeared in a Sydney court today on charges of assault, assault occasioning actual bodily harm and resisting arrest.

Chairman of the SCG Trust, Mr Pat Hills, said today he would discuss with police a total ban on alcohol to try to prevent a repetition of last night's rioting.

**Figure 6.1:** From the *Telegraph*, 15 January 1986.

sport – spectator violence. The policewoman blames abuse of alcohol for the violence.

Alcohol abuse has often been identified as a major cause of spectator misbehaviour and, in some places, spectators are not allowed to take alcohol into the sports ground. Nevertheless, alcohol is often served inside the grounds. Some people argue that alcohol should be banned entirely from sporting venues. They claim that there is no need for alcohol at sporting functions. Others argue that banning alcohol is unfair to the many who wish to have a drink and who cause no trouble; in addition, they point out that sales of alcohol help pay for sporting equipment and facilities. Individual violence, however, is not the greatest concern. Crowd violence which can and has

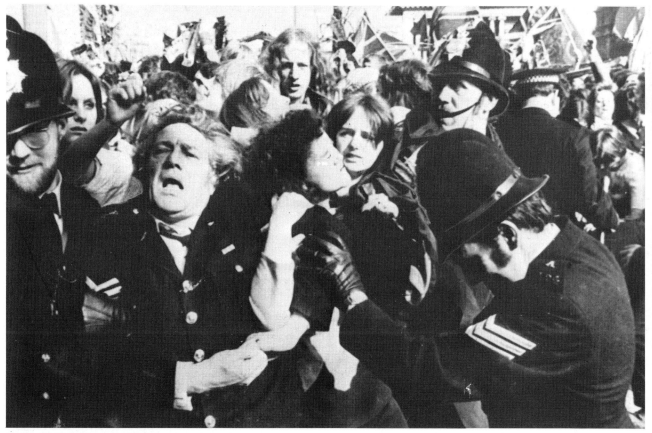

Police often have to bear the brunt of crowd violence.

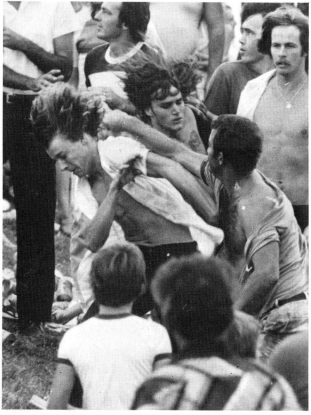

Individual violence.

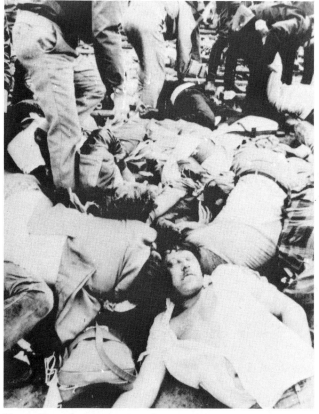

The ultimate tragedy of crowd violence.

led to multiple deaths, as witnessed in the 1985 soccer riots in Belgium, is of concern all around the world. Many different reasons have been suggested for large-scale crowd violence:

- The abuse of alcohol before entering and while at the grounds.
- The acceptance of violence by many fans. They have grown up with it, and many consider it a normal part of behaviour.
- The intense loyalty of fans who work themselves up to fever pitch over the results of matches.
- The noise and excitement. Some feel that the chanting of thousands in unison has the effect of heightening crowd excitement and aggression.
- Abnormal behaviour. Psychologists claim that some individuals in large crowds behave aggressively in ways not normal to them because they feel part of the crowd and therefore no longer individually responsible for their actions.
- Aggression towards opposing spectators. It is claimed some groups of spectators see opposing fans as "enemies". They do not see them as individual sports lovers but as a group to be insulted, heckled or even attacked.
- The economic situation of the fans. It is claimed that some fans who live in poorer conditions express their general frustration with life through violence.

Whatever the reason for spectator violence, it has an undesirable effect on sport and society.

- Countries whose citizens cause crowd violence gain a bad reputation as reports and photos of violence disgust and horrify people around the world.
- Individuals suffer injury, maiming or even death.
- Costs increase as safety fences are erected and police are paid to be present; shopkeepers have to fix broken windows; trains carrying spectators have to be repaired; costly court cases have to be arranged.

Apart from all this, a particular sport can suffer from the consequences of crowd violence. Gate takings depend on fans attending matches, and people who dislike violence stay away. Parents who wish to keep their children safe begin to direct them into sports where there is little crowd violence or even away from sport to other activities.

Spectator violence is a problem that most people want solved so that sport can flourish and spectators can enjoy the sport.

# Sponsors

As sport becomes a major form of entertainment, more and more media coverage takes place – the news has a sporting segment, newspapers allow 5 to 20 per cent of their space for sport, and radio and television devote enormous amounts of broadcasting time to it. Certain sports draw large audiences, and large audiences attract sponsors who wish to advertise their products.

Sponsors pay individuals and teams to wear their products, provide cash or prizes for sporting matches or pay for the coverage of a sporting contest on television. Sponsorship has had several effects, including:

- the growth of income among sporting stars
- the increasing cost of buying media rights; for example, the fees for televising the Olympic Games jumped from £260 000 in Rome in 1960 to £110 million for the Moscow Olympics in 1980. The American Broadcasting Corporation paid £100 million for the right to cover the 1984 Los Angeles Olympics and £135 million for the 1988 Calgary Winter Olympics. The media fees are one of the biggest funders of the Games.
- the demand that a sport become more marketable; for example, tie-breakers have been introduced to make tennis more exciting, and one-day cricket with

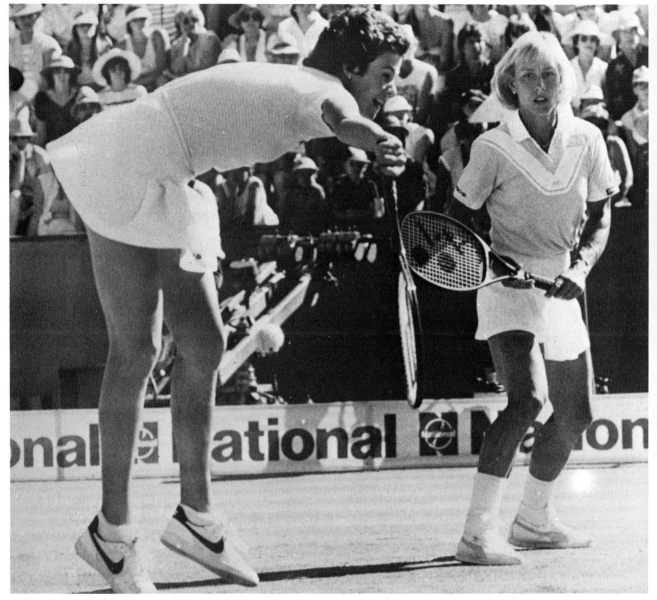

At the National Panasonic tennis classic. Note the sponsorship signs.

amended rules and colourful uniforms was introduced.

- the improvement in techniques of filming sport, e.g. the placement of cameras in racing cars and lightweight cameras on hang gliders.
- argument over sponsorship. Cigarette advertising is banned on television. Many people object to cigarette companies sponsoring sport, claiming that this indirectly advertises smoking and links cigarettes with sport; others argue that sporting bodies should be able to accept sponsorship as they choose.

## Commentators

As sport has a large audience, the role of the radio and television commentators has grown in importance. Some commentators are known around the world and receive letters from different countries, some from fans, others from enthusiasts asking questions about the history of the sport. Many commentators are former sports stars who switched to the commentary box when their sporting career ended. Computer technology allows them to have information about sporting records at their fingertips.

# Other issues in sport

## Professionalism

A professional is a person who earns money from sport. Professionals can now make millions from their sport, not only by winning cash prizes but also by advertising products. Many have managers to organise this for them and to invest their money.

Widespread professionalism is a modern development in sport. At the turn of the century, sport was largely amateur and great effort was made to keep it so. Some people still argue that professionalism is bad for sport. They believe sport should be played for fun, not money. Others, however, point out that professional athletes are simply getting paid for their particular talent which often lasts for only a short period of their life. Staying at the top of a sport is not a lifetime possibility, for the body cannot keep up peak performance in middle age. Supporters of professional sport point out that top musicians, writers and artists can earn huge amounts from their talents and feel that those with sporting talent should also be able to make money. They also believe that professionalism has brought higher standards of performance to sport.

This argument between those who support amateur sport and those who accept professional sport has affected the Olympic Games. The Games are restricted to amateurs. Today, there is increasing pressure to open the Games to professionals, not only to bring the high level of skill of professionals to Olympic competition but also because it is increasingly difficult to distinguish between amateur and professional. Some countries accept sports stars into the army where they can train uninterrupted. Individuals can advertise and attract money because of their superstar status, although the money has to be placed in a trust fund until they give up their amateur status. Educational scholarships are available which allow students to train without other commitments. Yet all these athletes are officially classed as amateurs in international competition.

Professionalism has affected not only the top levels of sport but also the grassroots level of sport in local clubs; for example, some local football teams pay bonuses for goals scored. No longer do many individuals expect to pay the major costs of training for their sports. They expect subsidies or the provision of expensive equipment.

## Sport and politics

When sport becomes involved in politics and foreign affairs the British population splits in its attitude, some arguing that sport and politics should not be mixed, and others arguing that it is impossible for them not to be. A recent example was the controversy over South African-born Zola Budd and whether she should have been issued with a British passport in order for her to compete for Great Britain.

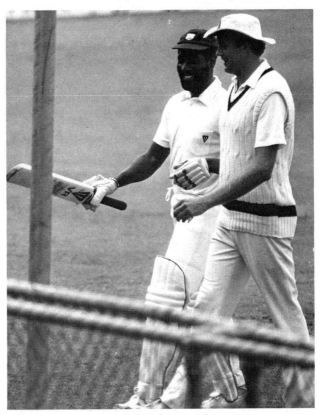

Sport can bring nations closer together.

# Conflict over sport and politics

When the Olympics were held in Moscow in 1980, the British Goverment asked sportsmen and women not to take part, but individuals were allowed to make up their own minds. This was a protest against the Russian military presence in Afghanistan. Although Britain was represented, some Sports Associations decided not to send teams. The British people were split in their opinions on the issue.

Many argued that politics had no place in sport and that the athletes should go to Moscow to compete. Others said that it is impossible to separate sport from politics and that the athletes should not go. Some countries, including the U.S.A., made a government decision that their athletes should not compete in Moscow.

The same kind of conflict exists over sporting contacts with South Africa. The South African government has been accused of denying civil rights to black South Africans. Because of this, pressure from around the world has been placed on nations to isolate South Africa until its government changes its views. Many nations have agreed not to send teams to South Africa and to refuse South African teams the right to tour their countries. Further, some nations are prepared to boycott sporting events run by countries which allow sporting contact with South Africans. Thus, sport has become a weapon of foreign policy.

The British government takes the view that there should be no official sporting contact between the two countries. Some Britons support this stand because they feel that the South African apartheid system is wrong. Some, however, support sporting contact with South Africa claiming that it is absurd to single out South Africa when we play against other nations also accused of denying rights to their citizens.

Other people believe that sport is sport and should not be connected with political decisions. They also point out that if the government were serious in its attitude to apartheid, it would cut all links, including trade, and not expect only sports people to apply bans.

# Sport and terrorism

At the Munich Olympics in 1972, some Israeli athletes and officials were murdered by terrorists. The world was outraged, and since that time countries hosting international events have feared a repetition of terrorism and have had to increase their security measures. This means the use of police and military forces, which increases the cost of holding large sporting events, restricts freedom of movement of athletes, press and spectators, increases the tension of organisers and lessens the friendly atmosphere.

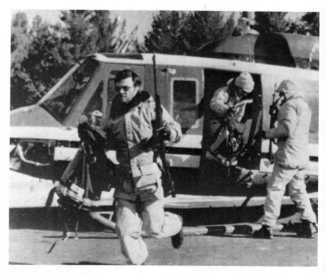

Tight security measures are now part of the Olympic Games.

# Sport and women

Women have always participated in a great range of sports.

Unfortunately, this has not always been recognised by the media or society.

Both physiological and sociological factors have influenced women's participation in sport at all levels. Before the age of 11, boys and girls can compete on equal terms, it is not until after adolescent development that anatomical differences makes equal competition between the sexes harder to achieve. These differences are exemplified in bone structure and muscle development.

In terms of performance when men's and women's world records are compared the men's records are better, but in some events the difference between the records has become less. The swimming records set by Mark Spitz in 1968 were broken by women ten years later. This narrowing of differences is particularly true in endurance events such as long distance swimming, running and cycling. Women are achieving these performances in events such as marathon running because they burn body fats more efficiently than men. In Cross Channel swimming women have an advantage with their more extensive covering of fat as it assists in sustaining body temperature and helps to maintain a good body position.

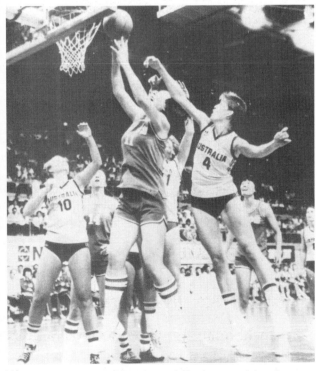

Women can now represent their countries in their own basketball teams.

Apart from these physiological factors, there are other reasons why women's performances have radically improved. For instance, it is more socially acceptable for women to train and devote a great deal of their life to sport. By having greater access to training facilities and improved training methods women over the last two decades have been able to attain a higher level of performance.

Women have many roles to fulfil in society: housewife, mother and often wage earner. This has sometimes made it difficult for women to be involved regularly in sport. With the development of Sports and Leisure Centres, more activities have been provided for women. Sports organisers have recognised the unique position of women and have begun to provide crèches, activities at off-peak times, concessionary rates, sports that particularly attract women such as aerobics, and "women-only" activities.

Today, although sports media coverage still favours men, there is increasing attention being paid to women in sport. Female sports stars are as much household names as male stars, and there are more women sports commentators. Television coverage of the Olympic Games has increased respect for female athletes and brought them into the limelight.

## Women and the Olympics

The involvement of women in sport and the changing attitude of society can best be seen in women's participation in Olympic events. Baron Pierre de Coubertin described women's involvement in the Olympic Games as "a very unedifying spectacle for the spectators". No doubt it was attitudes such as this that meant that only six women took part in the Paris Games in 1900, and competed in only two sports: tennis and golf.

Slowly the numbers of competitors rose and women's events were added to the

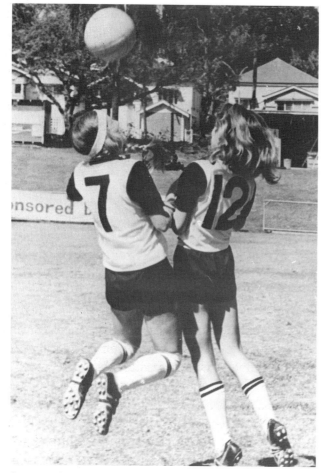

Soccer is now being enjoyed by females.

# Sport and disabled people

The aims of sport encompass the same principles for disabled people as they do for the able-bodied. In addition, for disabled people, sport has an immense therapeutic value and plays a great part in physical, psychological and social rehabilitation.

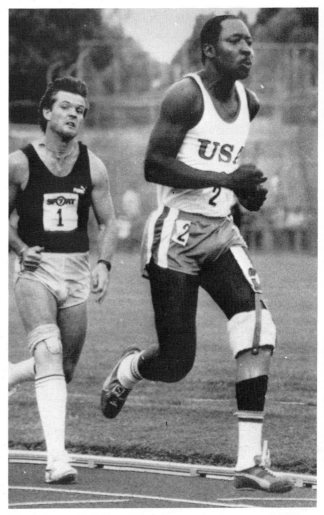

An international 100-metre race for amputees.

Olympic programme. By the Los Angeles Olympics in 1984 there were 75 events that women could take part in.

One of the most controversial areas was long distance running. It was not until 1960 that women were allowed to run further than 200 metres as the I.O.C. (International Olympic Committee) thought that long distance running did not suit women. Now women compete in races of all distances including marathons.

Today, there are opportunities for women to participate in almost any sport. As society's attitude changes, families become smaller, leisure time increases and more women become financially independent, it is hoped that with the encouragement of the media and organisations such as the Health Education Authority and the Sports Council the level of participation and involvement in sport will continue to increase.

The severity of a person's handicap and how much their equilibrium has been affected determines their training and participation in sport. With new technology most games can be adapted for disabled people and rules may be modified to accommodate the nature of a disability.

The attitude of society towards disabled people has been negative until the last few decades. It was not until World War II, which left thousands of people disabled, that a major initiative was taken up to help disabled people. In 1944 the Disabled Person's Employment Act was passed. This act improved the attitude of society towards disability.

In July 1948, the Stoke Mandeville Games were founded by Sir Ludwig Guttman, as an annual sports festival for the paralysed. The Games took place on the day the Olympic Games started in London, showing the public that sport was not the privilege of the able-bodied. These Games have continued to develop for all disabled people and every four years they are held in the same country as the Olympic Games.

When designing new sports facilities consideration is now given to the needs of disabled people. To allow them greater access facilities such as ramps, lifts, adequate changing areas and, deck-level swimming pools have been included along with access to social and refreshment areas. There are three main categories of activities and sport which disabled persons can take part in:

- those in which they compete on equal terms with little or no modification, e.g. bowls or archery.
- existing sports modified, e.g. wheelchair basketball.
- sports activities designed specifically for disabled people, e.g. goalball for the visually impaired.

Integration of disabled people into sporting activities has led to their inclusion in events such as the London Marathon. Other events which have assisted integration include the United Nation's Year of Disabled People and the Sports Council campaign Sport for All – Disabled People. Nevertheless, a great deal remains to be done before the slogan "Sport for All" achieves its full meaning.

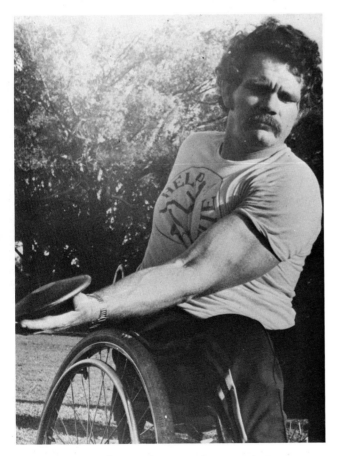

Many disabled people spend enormous amounts of time preparing for athletic events.

# Drugs and sport

A few athletes, constantly trying to improve their performance, have taken "short cuts". One short cut has been to use various drugs. In fact, many of the drugs used have not produced the desired improvement; on the contrary, they have led to long-lasting, irreparable body damage and on some occasions even to death. For example, Danish cyclist Knut Jensen died in a cycling event at the 1960 Olympics in Rome; English cyclist Tommy Simpson died during the 1967 Tour de France. Both had been using stimulants in an attempt to boost their performances.

Authorities are concerned about this problem for two main reasons:
- the damage to athletes who, more than most people, should value their health
- the unfair advantage that could arise from the use of drugs.

In major sporting events, tests are now used to identify athletes using drugs and to disqualify them from competition. Authorities continue to try to eliminate the use of drugs in sports by educating players, coaches and officials in the very real dangers of the use of drugs.

# Changing views

You have seen that there have been great changes in sport – in ethics, professionalism, media attitudes, and political pressures. However, there are other changing views too.

- Some people argue that we must find less aggressive ways to live. They condemn sport as encouraging unhealthy competition and aggression. They argue that the emphasis on contest should be ended and that people should be encouraged to participate in recreation where there are no winners or losers but simply people cooperating to enjoy themselves.
- Some people argue that schools should not organise competitive sport because of the stress on students, the emphasis on winning and the different size and maturity levels of students.

However, many people still believe that sport is a healthy pastime that builds character and cooperative team work. They believe students should be encouraged to participate in sport.

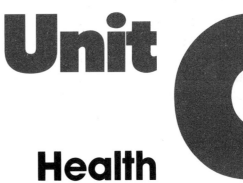

## The health revolution

In the last twenty years, there have been such great changes in attitudes towards health that we talk about a "health revolution". Because of this "health revolution", many people today are more aware of health as an important part of their lives. They are better informed about health, and increasingly are taking action to improve their health.

Signs of the health revolution are all around you: there are people jogging, cycling, and working out in gyms, and many books have been published on health, diet, nutrition, stress and relaxation. The Health Education Authority has taken a great interest, with campaigns such as the "Looking After Yourself" programme, and by providing funds for recreation and sport.

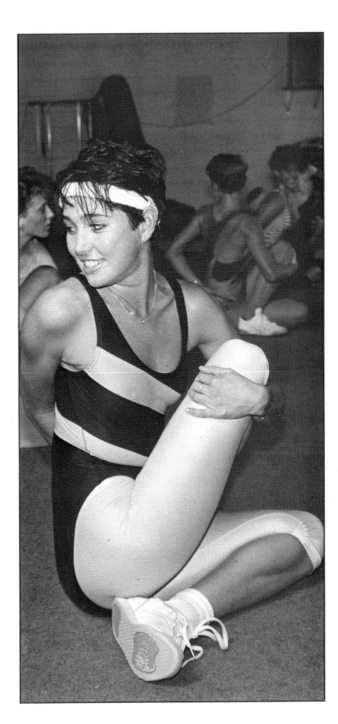

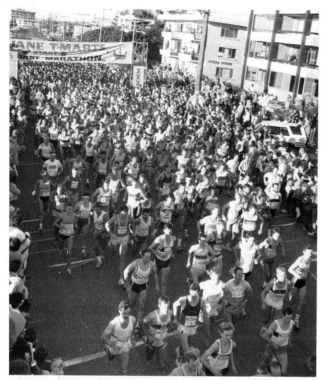

More and more people are joining in "fun runs". It is still very important to train before entering such events, even if you intend to run for fun and not for competition.

The health revolution has come about for several reasons:

- *The explosion of knowledge.* Scientific advances in medicine especially have provided us with increased knowledge about the body.
- *Longer life.* People live longer owing to improved medical procedures and they want to remain active in their later years.
- *Higher standard of living.* Many people have more money to spend on a wider range of food, medical care and leisure.
- *Change in lifestyle.* Many people live in cities and work in offices that limit physical activity. This, combined with rich food and labour-saving devices, increases the risk of heart trouble. Many people, therefore, are taking more responsibility for their health and are realising that some form of exercise will benefit them enormously.

The health revolution, then, has encouraged people to make decisions about their health.

## Encouraging you to take part

In Britain the Health Education Authority and the Sports Council have run various campaigns and programmes to encourage people of different ages to take part in sport.

In the 1970s the, then, Health Education Council ran a programme called "Looking After Yourself". The booklets and materials helped individuals to assess their level of fitness, and then encouraged them to adopt a healthy diet balanced with a sensible exercise programme.

## Health Education Authority

The Sports Council began their "Sport for All" Campaign in 1972 which addressed the problems of a lack of facilities as well as encouraging individuals to take part. Even into the 1990s the Sports Council is still encouraging people to take part in sport.

From the initial "Sport for All" campaign other programmes followed, such as "Sport for All the Family". In 1981 the United Nations held the International Year of Disabled People. Alongside this the Sports Council began their "Sport for All – Disabled People" campaign, concentrating on increasing opportunities for disabled people to take part in sport and to enjoy sport for its own sake.

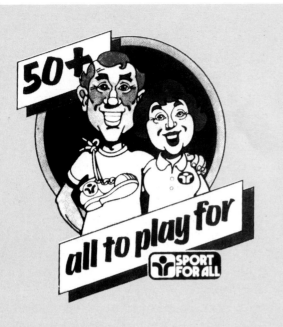

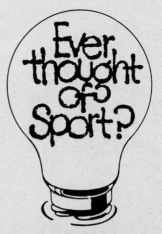

launched its "Ever Thought of Sport?" campaign in 1985.

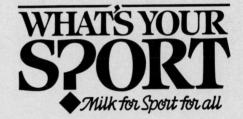

Encouraging the older person to take part in sport was the Council's next campaign. It was called "Fifty Plus – All to Play For" (1983). The information leaflets encouraged health check-ups and gave examples of sports that could be tried. Most importantly the leaflets said "playing's better than watching" to tempt the older person to take part in active sport.

Research by the Sports Council and other bodies has shown that children begin to drop out of sport towards the end of their school days. For many reasons, girls drop out more than boys at this age. To entice the 13–24 year-olds back to sport the Sports Council

More recently, the Milk Marketing Board has joined with the Sports Council in a campaign called "What's Your Sport?".

Whatever the slogan, the important factor is to encourage everyone to consider taking part in some form of active sport or recreation and adopt a healthy lifestyle.

# 7

# Health and you

## What is health?

In the past, health meant simply not being sick. However, the health revolution has meant that today we think of health as being much more than this. The components of health are:
- a feeling of physical well-being
- a feeling of mental and emotional well-being
- a feeling of social well-being
- the absence of illness and disease.

## Physical well-being

A feeling of physical well-being is usually achieved by:
- eating wisely
- seeking medical help when you are ill
- getting enough sleep
- having time for relaxation
- being physically fit.

## What is physical fitness?

People differ in their opinions about what physical fitness means. For some, it is being able to go about their everyday business without physical discomfort; for a top athlete, it is having a body tuned to peak performance. Not many of us are going to be or even want to be top athletes. Thus, for most of us, physical fitness for health means:

- having our body systems work efficiently
- being able to move with ease and enjoyment
- being able to maintain physical activity for extended periods without becoming fatigued.

## Why be fit?

Doctors have found that, compared with unfit people, fit people:
- have better-functioning body systems
- have less risk of heart disease
- have fewer ulcers
- have fewer muscular or joint aches
- develop fewer serious diseases
- recover faster from illness
- have a greater ability to cope with stress and emotional problems
- get tired less easily
- enjoy a greater variety of activities, many of which widen their circle of friends and enrich their lives.

Being fit has a beneficial effect on your body systems:
- *The cardio-vascular system.* Fitness increases the strength of the heart. Fit people tend to have hearts that beat more slowly, lessening the strain on this vital organ over a lifetime. Their blood vessels are usually in better condition, which increases the supply of blood to muscle and tissue, thus increasing the body's food supply and creating energy and endurance.

- *The respiratory system.* Fit people tend to have stronger muscles to aid the lungs, thereby increasing oxygen supply to the body.
- *The muscular system.* All muscles perform better in fit people, giving them greater endurance, strength, agility, and better functioning of the digestive and other systems.

# Becoming physically fit

More people are making the decision to become physically fit. However, if you are not fit, you should always consult a doctor before you undertake a fitness programme. Perhaps the doctor may want you to lose or gain weight before you start. If overweight, underweight or unfit people begin vigorous exercise programmes, they could injure themselves.

In fitness for health, there are two main factors to consider:
- having fun
- exercising suitably.

Exercising for health should be enjoyable. So choose exercises that are fun for you. If you are a person who enjoys company, exercise with friends. You can plan your exercise so that it doesn't become boring and your life doesn't become ruled by an exercise programme. Vary your activities so that you remain interested. You might consider some of the following ideas:
- *Water recreation.* Swim, canoe, windsurf, walk through the water parallel to the beach for 10 minutes.

- *Sports.* Join a club – tennis, badminton, cricket, rugby, football, squash, hockey.
- *Outdoor.* Jog, go for long walks, join an orienteering group, join an athletics group.
- *Cycle.* Cycle with a group of friends and enjoy the countryside at the same time.
- *Gym work.* Become a regular at a gym and ask the instructors to plan a programme with you.
- *Dancing.* Dancing is an excellent and enjoyable exercise. Go to discos or join a ballet, tap or jazz dance class.
- *Aerobics.* Join an aerobics class.

When you select your programme, always remember:
- Before starting exercise, you must warm up. At the end of the exercise, you should cool down.
- Never exhaust yourself. Danger signs are severe breathlessness, tightness or pain in the chest, nausea, the feeling you are losing control over your body. Stop immediately if these signs are present.
- Build up slowly according to your level of fitness. If you haven't been playing sport, don't hurry into an advanced training session. You'll only hurt yourself and learn to dislike exercise.
- Exercise regularly. To get the best value from exercise, you should exercise for at least 20 minutes from three to five times a week. It is even better if you can exercise for longer than 20 minutes, but stop if you feel fatigued. Don't decide that you should be fit and exercise madly every day for two weeks and then do nothing until your next guilty burst.
- You have to give your body time to recover from exercise. You can do this by having a lay-off or an easy exercise time every second day, and by getting plenty of sleep.

# 8

# Health and diet

Articles on food and diet can be found in many magazines and newspapers, all with different claims. Some claim that a particular diet or type of food can give people better health, control weight, improve performances, increase life expectancy and/or produce better skin. It is hard for people who are not nutrition experts to judge these claims, and sometimes time, effort and money can be wasted on something that has little value or benefit. Most authorities recommend eating a balanced diet. To understand how to achieve a balanced diet, you need to know about nutrients and the foods which contain them.

## What are nutrients?

Nutrients are those chemical substances in foods that are essential for the proper functioning of your body. Nutrients are vital for health, because they:
- enable the cells of the body to function efficiently
- help the body systems to function
- enable the body to grow
- help repair the body after illness or injury
- help prevent disease
- affect mental development.

## Nutrients in your diet

The essential nutrients in your diet include:
- carbohydrates
- proteins
- fats
- vitamins
- minerals.

In addition to these nutrients, you also need water and fibre.

## Carbohydrates

Carbohydrates are very important to a healthy diet. There are two types:
- Simple carbohydrates, which are sugars found in cane sugar, honey, fruit and milk. These are absorbed quickly into the bloodstream.
- Complex carbohydrates, which are mainly starches found in potatoes and cereals. Cereal products such as bread and pasta are therefore good sources of complex carbohydrates. Complex carbohydrates are absorbed more slowly into the bloodstream.

### Functions of carbohydrates

Carbohydrates:
- provide up to 70 per cent of the body's energy. They also provide heat. Complex carbohydrates are a good source of long-term energy.
- act as a protein sparer which means that, if your diet has adequate carbohydrate content, the protein does not need to be used to provide energy.
- are converted to fat and deposited around the body, especially under the skin, if they are eaten in excess.

# Proteins

Proteins make up a major part of all body cells, tissues and systems of the body including the hair, skin, muscle, bone and nerve fibre. Proteins are made up of amino acids. In the digestive system, protein is broken down into its amino acids and absorbed. There are about 23 amino acids. The body can manufacture many of these but there are nine essential amino acids which can be provided only by eating food containing them. Foods such as meat, milk, fish, eggs and soya beans contain these amino acids. People who don't eat meat must ensure they get all nine essential amino acids. This can be done by eating grains and pulses.

## Functions of proteins

Proteins:
- provide the amino acids which are required for the growth and repair of body cells and for some hormones and enzymes.
- provide the amino acids required for the formation of haemoglobin in the blood.
- provide energy and heat, although this is mostly the job of carbohydrates.

# Fats and oils

Fats and oils are essential for good health. There are three types of fats:
- *Saturated fats* which, when eaten excessively, raise blood cholesterol levels. This is believed to be a factor contributing to heart disease. These fats are found in meat, butter, dripping, coconut oil, chocolate, potato crisps and fried foods.
- *Mono-unsaturated fats* which do not affect cholesterol levels. They are found in olives, nuts (except walnuts) and avocados.

- *Polyunsaturated oils* which, some believe, tend to lower cholesterol levels. These are found in walnuts, fish oils, safflower and sunflower seeds, and soya beans.

Because of the large number of kilojoules contained in fat molecules, people who eat too much fatty food are more likely to gain weight. Being overweight can be a contributing factor to heart disease.

## Functions of fats

Fats:
- are a concentrated source of energy
- help absorb fat-soluble vitamins A, D, E and K
- help protect and support some organs of the body
- are found in the nerve sweat glands and glands of the skin
- are essential to good health.

# Vitamins

Vitamins are chemical compounds. They are essential to health but are required in minute quantities only. Vitamins play an important role in the healthy development of bones, skin and glands. Nutrition experts advise that a balanced diet contains all the vitamins necessary for a healthy life and advise against taking vitamin pills unless prescribed by a doctor. Overdoses of some vitamins can be poisonous.

Vitamins are divided into two main groups according to how they are absorbed in the body:
- fat-soluble vitamins – A, D, E and K
- water-soluble vitamins – all the B vitamins (often called B complex) and vitamin C.

Tables 8.1 and 8.2 summarise the vitamins, their sources and their functions.

**Table 8.1:** Water-soluble vitamins

| Vitamin | Source | Stability | Function | Deficiency problems |
|---|---|---|---|---|
| B1 (Thiamin) | Wheatgerm, yeast, wholegrain bread, pork, liver, eggs, brown rice, potatoes | Stable but destroyed by high temperatures | • Normal functioning of nervous system<br>• Needed so that carbohydrates can be used in the body | • Tiredness<br>• Loss of appetite<br>• Loss of muscle tone |
| B2 (Riboflavin) | Milk, cheese, liver, eggs, wheatgerm, vegetables, kidney | Destroyed by sunlight; milk left in sunlight for two hours loses 50% of B2 | Needed for general health, healthy skin and eyes | Cracking at corners of mouth, sore tongue, itching of eyes |
| B3 (Niacin) | Fish, meat, wholemeal cereals, peanuts, legumes, yeast | Destroyed by over cooking | • Healthy skin<br>• Helps release of energy to the body<br>• Essential for growth | Few problems but extended deficiency may cause weakness, headache, loss of appetite |
| B5 (Pantothenic acid) | Liver, meat, eggs, fish, fresh vegetables | Destroyed by high temperatures and excessive freezing | • Involved in formation of red blood cells<br>• Needed so that protein, fat and carbohydrates can be used in the body | Few problems |
| B6 (Pyridoxine) | Meat, liver, wholegrain cereals, peanuts, eggs, soya beans | Stable, although destroyed by high temperatures | • Formation of red and white blood cells<br>• Needed so that protein can be used in the body | Few problems |
| B12 (Cyanocabalamin) | Liver, kidney, milk, pork, beef, seafood, cheese | Destroyed by high temperatures | Development of red blood cells | Anaemia |
| B (Folic acid) | Green vegetables, liver, kidney | Easily destroyed — vegetables need to be eaten raw | • Development of red blood cells<br>• Needed so that protein can be used in the body | Anaemia |
| B (Biotin) | Liver, yeast, nuts, beans, fish, eggs; found in smaller amounts in grains and vegetables | Stable | Needed so that fat and proteins can be used by the body | Very rare |
| C (Ascorbic acid) | Citrus fruits, green vegetables, potatoes | Easily destroyed by light, chopping, heat, salting | • Produces a substance that helps cement the tissues of the skin, bones and blood vessels<br>• Helps in the absorption of iron<br>• Helps wounds to heal<br>• Helps the body resist infection<br>• Helps normal growth in children<br>• Plays a role in red blood cell formation | • Slow healing<br>• Decreased resistance to infection<br>• Bleeding gums<br>• Excessive deficiency causes scurvy<br>• Bottle-fed babies who are not given orange juice or a source of vitamin C may get anaemia |

**Table 8.2:** Fat-soluble vitamins

| Vitamin | Source | Stability | Function | Deficiency problems |
|---|---|---|---|---|
| A | Liver, milk, butter, eggs, vegetables, fish | Very stable, although some loss at high temperature and long exposure to light | • Normal growth of children, especially of bones<br>• Maintains healthy skin and eyes<br>• Allows good vision in dim light | • Stunted growth<br>• Night blindness<br>• Rough skin |
| D | Sunlight on skin, milk, cheese, eggs, fishliver oils, liver | Very stable, not easily destroyed | Essential for strong healthy bones and teeth | Rickets |
| E | Vegetables, wheatgerm, nuts, eggs, vegetable oils | Not easily destroyed, although deep frying causes some destruction | Not fully understood, although it helps in maintaining a healthy muscular and vascular system | Few problems. It is more common for people to suffer from excess owing to taking vitamin pills. |
| K | Green vegetables, soya beans, liver, fruit, fish | • Not destroyed by steam cooking<br>• Destroyed by light | Important in blood clotting | • Slow blood clotting<br>• Bleeding (haemorrhage) in infants |

# Minerals

Minerals account for only 6 per cent of total body weight but they are essential for normal development. They play a vital role in all body processes. The body contains many minerals, some in relatively large quantities, others in minute amounts. Our knowledge of minerals and their functions is still incomplete. Some minerals exist in such minute amounts that they are very difficult to study.

Table 8.3 summarises the minerals and their functions. As chlorides, magnesium phosphorus and sulphur are present in quantity in most foods and do not present a dietary problem, we have not included them in the table.

# Water and fibre

In addition to the nutrients, a balanced diet must include:
● water
● fibre (roughage).

# Water

Water makes up about 60 per cent of your body weight. You should drink about 5–6 medium-size glasses of water each day.

### Functions of water

Water:
● provides the moisture necessary for all living tissue except the nails, hair and teeth
● helps the chemical reactions in the body
● dilutes and moistens food
● dilutes waste products and poisonous substances in the body.

## Fibre

It is only recently that fibre has been identified as an essential part of a diet. Fibre is found in all plant cells. It is that part of a plant that cannot be entirely digested. The best sources of fibre are:
● nuts, seeds, legumes – chick peas, lentils, baked beans, nuts, seeds

**Table 8.3:** Minerals and their functions

| Mineral | Source | Some functions | Deficiency problems |
|---------|--------|----------------|---------------------|
| Sodium | Fish, meats, all manufactured foods, salt | • Sodium plus calcium strenthens bones<br>• Assists fluid movement in cells | Difficult to be deficient as many foods contain sodium |
| Potassium | Fish, meat, vegetables, citrus fruits, grapes | Important role in muscle contraction, especially the heart | • Only extremes of high and low concentration affect the body<br>• Low concentration can cause muscle weakness and abnormal heart beat<br>• a very high concentration can stop the heart |
| Calcium | Sardines, milk, cheese, eggs, creamed cottage cheese, salmon, green vegetables | • A major part of bones and teeth; especially important during their formation in a foetus and in childhood.<br>• Essential in blood clotting<br>• Nerve transmission and muscle contraction | • Muscle spasms<br>• Cardiac or respiratory failure<br>• Rickets |
| Iron | Liver, beef, shellfish, spinach, dried fruits, egg yolk, dark chocolate | Allows haemoglobin to carry oxygen into tissues | • Anaemia<br>• Fatigue, loss of efficiency, proneness to accidents |
| Iodine | Seafood, vegetables grown near the sea | • Helps body processes<br>• Essential to thyroid hormone | Goitre |
| Fluorine | • Found naturally in some drinking water<br>• Artificially added to water | • Strengthens teeth and bones<br>• Helps prevent tooth decay | Tooth decay |
| Zinc | Oysters, wheatgerm, cheddar cheese, wholewheat grain, lean roast beef | Participates in body processes | • Impaired growth of the foetus and infant<br>• Poor healing<br>• Loss of taste |
| Copper | Organ meats, shellfish, nuts, whole-grain cereals | • Enables correct functioning of some enzymes<br>• Essential for absorption of iron<br>• Maintains a healthy nervous system | Anaemia |

• whole cereals – brown rice, bread and spaghetti, unprocessed bran and muesli, oatmeal
• root vegetables – potatoes, parsnips, onions, carrots

• vegetables, fruit – all fruits, fresh and dried; all leafy vegetables.

Processed foods may not be good sources of fibre as sometimes the fibre is broken down in processing.

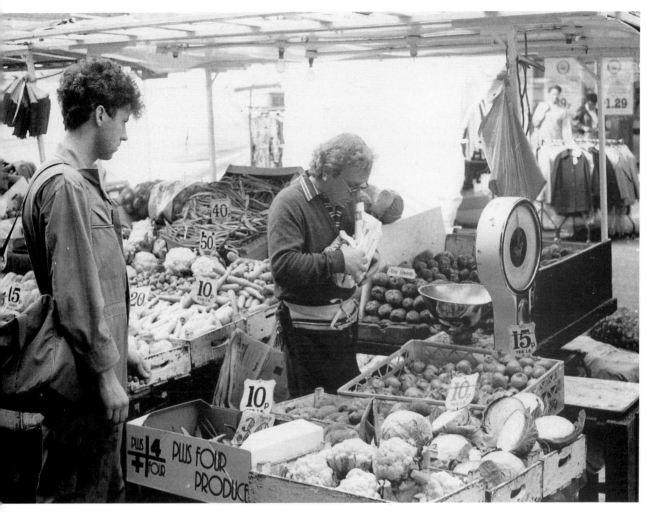

More people are including greater quantities of fruit and vegetables in their diet.

## Functions of fibre

Scientists have found a link between a diet low in fibre and a range of diseases. However, this does not mean that we can say that a deficiency can cause these diseases.

- Fibre creates a bulk in the intestine by absorbing many times its weight in water, thus making it easier to excrete waste from the body. A lack of fibre can lead to constipation.
- Some doctors claim that a diet low in fibre may increase the risk of cancer of the colon.
- Fibre found in soya beans, lentils, mung beans and spinach may play a part in lowering blood cholesterol levels by decreasing the absorption of fat and cholesterol from food.

"Balanced diet" is a term we use to describe a diet that contains each nutrient in the correct proportions. Of course, what makes a balanced diet depends on a number of factors, including:

- size – the amount of nutrients needed varies from person to person
- age – adolescence is a time when you are active and require high energy levels
- your level of activity.

Most of the foods you eat contain a number of nutrients; for example, potatoes and bread are good sources of carbohydrates, and they also contain some protein and vitamins. This means that if you eat a varied diet you are more likely to get all the nutrients you need.

# The six food groups

In order to achieve a balanced diet you need to have a certain amount of information about the foods available from which you can choose.

There are various ways of classifying food into groups. The food group system shown here was suggested in the Nutritional Guidelines issued by the Inner London Education Authority in 1985. This has been selected because of its simplicity and, unlike many other ways of grouping, can be used within a multi-cultural context.

Figure 8.1:

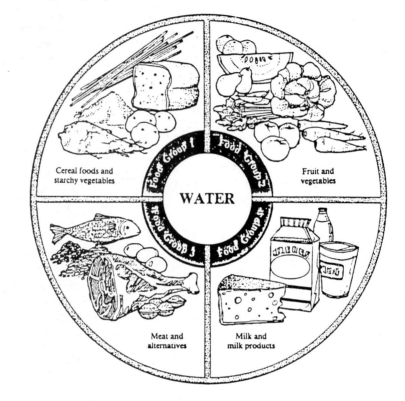

A daily diet which includes food from each of these groups is likely to be a healthy eating pattern. However, many animal foods are high in fat, so it is important to choose those with a lower fat content more frequently, e.g. white fish, chicken, lean meat, skimmed milk, low fat cheese.

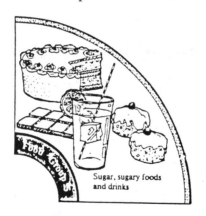

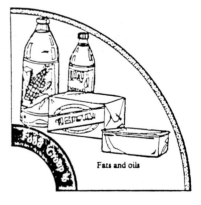

These foods add palatability, food energy and some polyunsaturated fatty acids to the diet. They should not, however, replace foods from the four main groups and their consumption should be limited.

# Water

Water is an important part of the diet and is needed to maintain the fluid balance of the body. Drinks fit easily into the food group system. Remember, water is also found in foods, especially fruit and vegetables.

# Healthy eating

Many nutritionists point out that some diets contribute to health problems including heart disease, obesity, high blood pressure, tooth decay and colon cancer. They suggest that your diet should:

- include foods from the five food groups.
- control weight by reducing fat, sugar and alcohol intake. Lean meats and low-fat dairy products are preferred, and food should be steamed rather than fried.
- contain less sugar and salt. Excessive sugar leads to tooth decay and obesity. Salt may contribute to high blood pressure. For this reason, it is recommended that no salt be added to food in cooking or for eating.
- include water rather than soft drink, cordials, tea or coffee.

These ideas are shown in Figure 8.2.

| EAT LEAST | sugar, butter, margarine, oil |
|---|---|
| EAT MODERATELY | milk, cheese, yoghurt, poultry, lean meat, nuts, eggs |
| EAT MOST | cereals, bread, vegetables, fruit |

**Figure 8.2:** A healthy approach to eating.

## Visible signs of nutrition

Doctors look for signs to indicate the possible health of a patient. They are careful to treat possible signs of poor nutrition only as clues as these may also be the result of poor hygiene, over-exposure to the sun, an infectious disease or lack of exercise.

| Part of body | Possible signs of good nutrition | Possible signs of poor nutrition |
|---|---|---|
| Hair | Shiny, healthy scalp | Dull, dry, brittle |
| Eyes | Bright, clear, moist | Dry, lack of shine, sunken, dark rings arounds eyes |
| Teeth | Clean, white, straight | Crooked, blackened |
| Gums | Pink, firm | Red around teeth, bleed easily |
| Face | Clear skin, healthy looking | Patchy skin, dark rings around eyes, sunken eyes |
| Muscles | Firm, good tone | Flabby, lack of tone, under-developed, |
| Stomach | Flat | Swollen |

# Weight control

Food provides the body with energy. As it is useful to know how much energy individual foods can provide when processed by the body, we use the unit of energy known as the joule. One thousand joules equal one kilojoule. We say that an apple has 200 kilojoules because it provides us with 200 kilojoules of energy. Foods do not contain the same amount of kilojoules per gram; for example, alcohol has 30 kilojoules per gram, fats have 37, but carbohydrates have only 16.

When you eat, you take in food which provides energy for activity. What is not used is stored as body fat. We can say:

$$\text{Energy taken in} = \text{Energy used} + \text{Energy stored (body fat)}.$$

Therefore, if you take in more energy than you use, you will put on weight. To lose weight, you must either decrease food intake or increase physical activity, or do both. Fad diets do not lead to long-term weight loss and may, in fact, be dangerous. Unless you are dieting under medical supervision, you should aim to lose only about a half to 1 kilogram per week by eating a well-balanced diet and increasing your physical activity.

### Stable weight

Energy taken in (food and drink) = Energy used (activity)

### Weight gain

Energy taken in > Energy used

### Weight loss

Energy taken in < Energy used

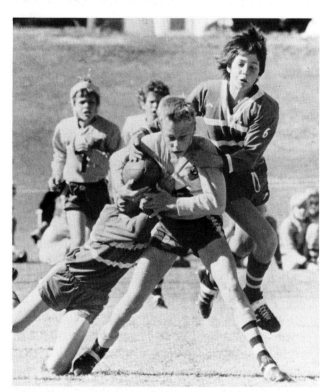

The more active you are the more kilojoules you use.

You do not need to be thin to be healthy. Look at the charts in Figure 8.3. You will see that your body mass can vary over a range of kilograms and still be well within the "healthy" range.

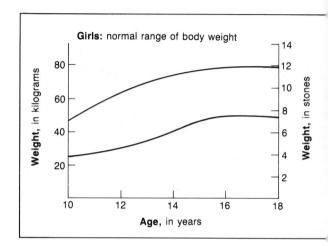

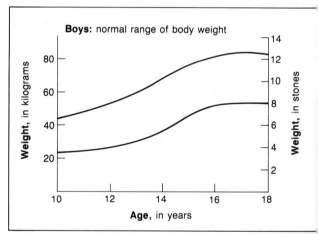

**Figure 8.3:** Normal weight ranges.

# 9

# Drugs and your health

## What are drugs?

Drugs are chemicals occuring in natural forms or made in laboratories which can alter normal functioning of the body in some way. They can affect a person's physical or emotional condition or both. Some drugs can even change mood and behaviour. In our society, some drugs are legal and some are not. Some drugs, when used medically, can be an aid to health, such as those prescribed by a doctor to fight illness and disease. Just because a drug is legal, however, does not necessarily mean that it is beneficial to your health. All drugs can be dangerous when abused, and abuse of drugs is one of the greatest health problems in our society. This chapter will concentrate on drugs not prescribed by doctors, in particular those drugs obtained through drinking and smoking.

## Smoking

Cigarettes contain the drug nicotine as well as tar and other dangerous chemicals. Smoking deposits tar into the lining of the lungs, and sends dangerous chemicals into the body. Smokers can become addicted to nicotine and find it difficult to give it up.

### Facts about cigarette smoking

- It takes 7.5 seconds for nicotine to reach the brain from the lungs.

- Tar contains chemicals which may help cause cancer in the mouth, throat and lungs.
- Nicotine speeds up the heartbeat, which causes you to be less relaxed and increases the risk of heart attack.
- Nicotine increases blood pressure by narrowing the blood vessels, which causes you to be more tense, again increasing the risk of heart attack.
- Smoking decreases the flow of blood and air in your lungs thus causing your lungs to be less effective.
- Smoking decreases the blood flow to your hands and feet, causing a decrease in skin temperature.
- Smoking damages taste buds on your tongue, and thus your senses of taste and smell are less sensitive.
- Smoking makes your breath, hair and clothes smell of stale smoke.
- Smoking causes your skin to wrinkle at an earlier age than normal.
- If pregnant women smoke, the chances are that the baby will be smaller than normal or may be premature, and the likelihood of infant death is increased.
- Atherosclerosis of the coronary arteries is more common in smokers than in non-smokers. Atherosclerosis cuts down the blood flow and causes the heart to work harder. If the arteries of the heart are affected, a heart attack can follow.
- Smoking damages the cilia in the bronchioles and lungs so that bacteria and other wastes cannot be removed. A

smoker's cough is an attempt to get rid of these waste products.

- Smoking makes it more likely that your bronchioles and lungs can become infected resulting in bronchitis.
- Smoking damages the air sacs of the lungs. This can result in emphysema. People with emphysema have difficulty breathing and very quickly lose their breath even during light exercise.
- Smokers have a much higher risk of gum disease.
- One person smoking in a room will affect the health and comfort of all the others in the room. People who do not smoke but live or work in the same area as a smoker may, over a long period of time, suffer the same ill-effects as the smoker.

**Towards a smoke-free generation**

In Britain there has been a campaign to tackle smoking by young people, especially girls. The programme began in 1985 and is scheduled to last five years.

**The extent of the problem**

- 100,000 people die prematurely each year from smoking related diseases.
- It is estimated that some 300,000 young people (125,000 boys, 175,000 girls) smoke at least one cigarette a week.
- Approximately one in seven 11-year-olds have experimented with cigarettes.
- From the age of 13 onwards more girls than boys are regular smokers.
- It is estimated that school children are sold some £10m worth of cigarettes, illegally, each year.

**Figure 9.1:** Percentage of regular smokers by age, 1988.

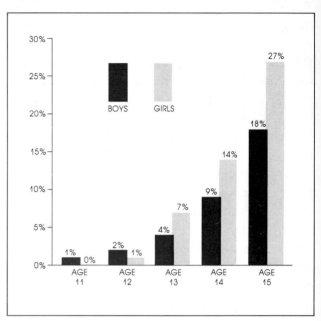

*Source:* E. Goddard: *Smoking among secondary school children in England, 1988* (H.M.S.O., 1989).

**What are the immediate dangers to children?**

Some smokers suffer while still at school. Children who smoke have an increased risk of suffering health problems such as bronchitis, ear, nose and throat infections, pneumonia and asthmatic attacks while still at school.

- Smokers are more frequently absent from school, are more likely to be under-achievers and to achieve lower grades overall than non-smokers.
- Young people become addicted to nicotine at an early age, but do not recognise their dependence until it is well established.

**Figure 9.2:** Smoking among fifth-year boys and girls in England, 1982–1988.

| Year | 1982 | | 1984 | | 1986 | | 1988 | |
|---|---|---|---|---|---|---|---|---|
| Regular smoker | 26% | 28% | 31% | 28% | 19% | 30% | 18% | 33% |
| Occasional smoker | 10% | 11% | 10% | 11% | 6% | 7% | 8% | 9% |
| Gender | ♀ | ♂ | ♀ | ♂ | ♀ | ♂ | ♀ | ♂ |

**Note**   Regular smoking is defined as usually smoking at least one cigarette a week.
Occasional smoking is defined as being a current smoker and smoking less than one cigarette a week.

*Source:* E. Goddard: *Smoking among secondary school children in England, 1988* (H.M.S.O., 1989).

# Drinking

Alcohol is a legal and commonly available drug. Alcohol abuse is the most common drug abuse in our society today. The majority of people use this drug for social occasions and can control the amount they drink. However, some people become addicted to alcohol and lose control of their lives. It must be remembered that it is illegal for a child under 18 to buy or drink alcohol in a public place.

Alcohol needs no digesting (breaking down). It passes through the walls of the stomach and small intestine into the bloodstream. It can be found in the blood minutes after a drink. This happens more quickly when:
- drinking strong drinks
- drinking fast
- drinking when hungry.

The alcohol in the blood is carried to all parts of the body. The effects of alcohol depend on:
- the amount of alcohol in the drink
- the number of drinks
- the weight of the drinker
- the time the body has to get rid of the alcohol.

The body gets rid of the alcohol through the liver. The liver takes nearly an hour to change the alcohol in one drink into energy.

There is about the same amount of alcohol in each of the drinks shown in figure 9.4. Alcohol will build up in the blood if more than one drink is taken in an hour. People will become drunk if they have too many drinks. Keep to the sensible limits if you want to avoid damaging your health. A unit is half a pint of beer, a glass of wine or a single measure of spirits.

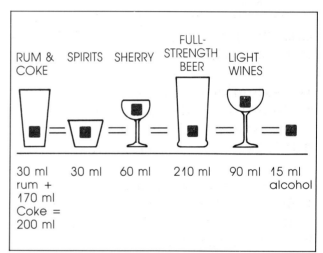

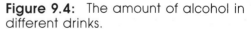

**Figure 9.4:** The amount of alcohol in different drinks.

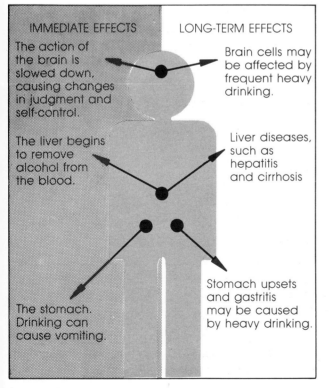

**Figure 9.3:** The effects of alcohol abuse on the body.

Drink can make some people lively and chatty, others silent and unsociable. It is worth remembering that alcohol is not a stimulant, despite what many people believe. It is a depressant in the sense that it depresses certain brain functions. That means it affects your judgement self-control and co-ordination.

| FOR MEN | FOR WOMEN |
|---|---|
| Up to 21 units a week | Up to 14 units a week |
| spread throughout the week, with 2 or 3 drink free days | |
| HOW MUCH IS TOO MUCH? | |
| FOR MEN | FOR WOMEN |
| 36 units or more in a week | 22 units or more in a week |
| if you drink as much as this or more then damage to your health is likely | |

**Figure 9.5:** Sensible drinking

## Possible long-term effects

The long-term effects of heavy drinking can be:
- stomach disorders
- depression
- vitamin deficiency
- sexual difficulties
- brain damage
- muscle disease
- hepatitis
- cirrhosis
- cancer of the mouth, throat and gullet
- more problems for people with diabetes.

## Facts about drinking

- Alcohol is a major cause of accidents.
- More than half the people breathalysed are over twice the legal limit.
- One in three of the drivers killed in road accidents have levels of alcohol which are over the legal limit.
- Most drinking and driving accidents, happen within one mile of the driver's home.
- Young people are affected more quickly by drinking than older people.

If you drink sensibly, you can prevent making a fool of yourself, damaging your health, having a hangover, becoming involved in an accident or hurting other people.

# Drugs

Drugs can mean everything from cigarettes to heroin. There is no single reason why anyone takes drugs. Most young people probably start simply from curiosity or because their friends are doing it. Others like taking risks, particularly if they know their parents or other adults would disapprove. Some may take drugs because they are bored and some because they are depressed or worried.

Probably the most powerful influence on whether you will smoke, drink or use illegal drugs is the pressure placed on you by friends and other people of your own age group. When it comes to drugs, this pressure can be very harmful. Work out your own attitude to all drugs.

In sport, performers have always taken various drugs in order to improve their performance. It is generally considered unfair and dangerous to use drugs to enhance performance, and athletes who are found to be using them are subject to harsh penalties. But in spite of the effects of national and international doping committees, some athletes and performers have continued to take drugs.

## Stimulants

Stimulants are used in sports where physical fitness is critical. They can improve and increase the work level of the athlete and delay fatigue.

The most widely used stimulants are amphetamines, first produced in 1887 and used to treat nervous diseases. One of the effects of this type of drug is a powerful feeling of well-being and confidence. It was also believed that they increased the physical capacity for strenuous tasks without destroying judgement.

In terms of endurance, amphetamines can prolong performance. When reaching the limits of endurance, pain is a warning for the body to stop before damage occurs. Football players taking amphetamines have been

**Table 9.1** Drugs and their effects

| Drug | Manner used | Physical dependence | Psychological dependence | Immediate after-effects | Mental complications | Physical complications | Results of overdose |
|---|---|---|---|---|---|---|---|
| Alcohol | By mouth | With exess usage | Yes | Confusion, delirious state | Intoxication | Gastritis, pancreatitis, cirrhosis, neuritis | Coma, respiratory failure |
| Amphetamines (stimulants) | By mouth and injection | Uncertain | Yes | Depression, aggressiveness, hallucinations | Hyperactivity, confusion | Liver and kidney damage, malnutrition, infection from needle | Convulsions, coma, brain haemorrhage |
| Barbiturates (sedatives) | By mouth and injection | Yes | Yes | Withdrawal, delirium, convulsions, confusion | Intoxication, confusion | Anxiety, nausea, slowed reactions | Coma, respiratory failure, shock |
| Cocaine | By mouth, inhalation, and injection | Yes | Yes | Depression, loss of coordination hallucinations | Hyperactivity, confusion | Malnutrition, perforated nose septum from sniffing | Convulsions, respiratory failure |
| Heroin | By mouth, inhalation and injection | Yes | Yes | Withdrawal — vomiting, diarrhoea, tremors, sweats, etc. | Intoxication | Infection from needle, anxiety, nausea, slowed reactions | Coma, respiratory failure |
| Marihuana | By mouth and inhalation | Unknown | Yes | Sometimes difficulty in concentration | Intoxication, (rare) panic | Heavy use — bronchitis, conjunctivitis, sometimes nausea | Death as a direct result of overdose is unknown |
| Minor analgesics (pain killers) | By mouth | None | Yes | None | None | Gastric ulcers, kidney failure, haemorrhage | Death has been known |
| Nicotine | By mouth | Yes (with high intake) | Yes | Sedation | None | Long-term heavy use — lung cancer, bronchitis, high blood pressure, heart disease | |

*Source:* Guest and Eshuys, *You Are a Citizen*, p. 64.

reported to have played on despite pain from injury. The dangers of continuing activity and suppressing pain could be pulled muscles, cramp and strains. Many believe that while there are physiological benefits, amphetamines only produce small improvements in some aspects of performance. Due to the effects of this drug, the British cyclist Tommy Simpson died of heart failure caused by heat exhaustion during the 1967 Tour de France. He was unable to recognize the point of exhaustion and continued to cycle.

The dosage of these stimulants must be steadily increased to improve the athlete's performance. The higher the dosage the greater the risk of suffering side-effects. It is possible to legislate and enforce regulations, because this type of drug can be traced in the urine.

## Anabolic steroids

Athletes attempting to enhance performance might take hormones or hormone substitutes such as anabolic steroids. Hormones are produced naturally in both males and females in varying quantities. Their purpose is to help repair the body after periods of physical stress and encourage growth and healing.

''Anabolic'' means ''building-up'' steroids are hormones. They have been used in sport to help develop athletes' power and speed up their recovery by artificially promoting muscle development.

Recent research has suggested that athletes who have taken anabolic steroids are able to train harder with less fatigue and require less recovery time. They seem not to have a direct effect on muscle bulk, but to enable the athlete to train at a more intensive level.

The side-effects of anabolic steroids can be divided into two categories, andronic and anabolic.

- Andronic effects include an increase of facial hair, lengthening of the vocal chords which causes the voice to "break", impotency and infertility.
- Whilst steroids make the athlete more competitive and aggressive, the anabolic side-effects include personality changes, early maturation of bone growth, and fluid retention.

By 1973, doctors were able to detect anabolic steroids, which led to the International Olympic Committee testing for the drugs at the Commonwealth Games. The first serious testing for anabolic steroids was carried out at the Montreal 1976 Olympics. Athletes realise that it takes more than two weeks to clear their bodies of all traces of steroids. Most testing at this time was restricted to major competitions. Today, random testing (that is testing of athletes at various stages of an event whether or not they win) has increased the possibility of drug use being detected.

## Pressures of sport

As athletes are forced to increase training loads, injuries caused by muscle over-use are a serious problem. Many athletes are unwilling to rest despite the pain and use pain killers instead.

Many young athletes have been forced to stop competing because they ignored the warning signs and took pain killers, thereby causing irreparable damage to their bodies.

# Index

**A**

abdomen injury, 112
adrenalin, 40
aerobic, 63, 64, 70, 71
alcohol, 1, 49–50
agility, 66, 85, 87
anabolic steroids, 151–152
anaerobic, 6, 63–4, 70, 72
anatomical position, 43–46
ankle injuries, 110
arteries, 27

**B**

balance, 51–54, 66
  improving, 87
bladder, 34, 35
blistering, 104
blood, 24, 28
  pressure, 27–28
  groups, 28
brain, 37–38
bruising, 105
burns, 104

**C**

carbohydrates
  for fitness, 92
  loading, 93
  in the diet, 138
cardio-vascular endurance, 64,
  68–69
  improving, 70, 87, 136
cartilage, 19
  injuries, 107–108
Cassius Clay (Mohammed Ali), 6
cells, 12, 13, 28
cerebellum, 37–38
chafing, 105
chest injury, 112
cholesterol, 139
choosing a sport, 97
circulatory system, 12, 19, 23
  functions of, 24
  structure and workings, 24–28,
    42
circuit training, 90–91
coaches, 121
Comaneci, Nadia, 9
commentators, 126, 129

continuous training, 90
cool-down, 91–92
Cooper, 12 minute run test, 68
coordination, 66, 67, 85
cork, 113
Coubertin, Baron Pierre de, 4, 5,
  129
cramp, 106

**D**

deceleration, 59
diaphragm, 30, 37
diet, 92, 138–146
digestive system, 12
  functions of, 31
  structure and workings of,
    32–34
disabled people and sport, 130–31
dislocation, 113
drinking (alcohol), 149–150
drugs, 135
  and their effects, 147, 150–51
  and sport, 131

**E**

ear injury, 111
elbow injuries, 110
endocrine system, 12, 38
  functions of, 38–39, 42
  structure and workings, 39–40
endurance, 64
ethics, 119
excretory system, 12, 34
  functions of, 34
  structure and workings, 34–35
eye injury, 111

**F**

fads and fallacies in fitness, 94
Fartlek training, 91
fats
  and fitness, 93
  in the diet, 139
feet and posture, 61
fibre, 141–43
fitness, 136–37
  and performance, 63
  components of, 63–67
  improving, 68–87, 137

flexibility, 65, 77
  assessing, 77–79
  improving, 80–83
food for fitness, 92
food groups, 144
footwear, protective, 100
force, 47
fractures, 108, 112
Fraser, Dawn, 9

**G**

games, 116, 117
glands, 39–40
gravity, 51–53
grazing, 104

**H**

haematoma, 113
hair, 41
hamstrings, 21
hard tissue injuries, 108
hard and easy days training, 89
Health Education Authority, 130,
  133, 134
health revolution, 133–35
health, 136–37
heart, 20, 26
  rate, 26, 70
heat exhaustion, 111
helmets, 100
hinge joint, 17, 43
history of sport, 2–3, 7–10
hitting the wall, 92
hormones, 39

**I**

Illinois agility run, 86
injuries, 95
  causes, 96–97
  prevention, 95–102
  treatments, 102–113
inspiration, 30–31
interval training, 90
intestines, 32–34
Isometrics, 77
Isotonics, 74

**J**

joints, 16–18
in movement, 42–43, 47–49
injuries, 109–10
judo, 49

**K**

Kasch-Boyer step test, 69
kidneys, 34–35
knee guards, 101
knee joint, 17
injuries, 109–10
Korbut, Olga, 6

**L**

laws of motion (Newton's), 55–57
levers, 47–50
Lewis, Carl, 10
ligament injuries, 107
lungs, 24, 29, 30–31

**M**

media and sport, 120, 126, 125
minerals, 93, 141
functions of, 142
motion and momentum, 54–58
mouthguards, 100
movement, 42–44
factors affecting, 47–57
types of, 44–46
muscles, 20, 42
injuries, 105–6
types of, 20–21
muscular system, 12, 19, 137
endurance, 64, 72–74, 87
functions of, 19, 42
structure and working, 19–23

**N**

nails, 41
nervous system, 2, 19, 35
functions of, 35, 42
structure and workings, 35–38
nose bleed, 111
Nurmi, Paava, 7–8
nutrients, 138–46
nutritional guidelines, 144–45

**O**

officials in sport, 121
Olympic Games, 2–10, 114
development of, 5–6, 125, 127,
129, 152
open wounds, 103

organised games, 114
organisers, sport, 122
overloading, 68, 89
Owens, Jesse, 8–9
oxygen debt, 72

**P**

padding, 101
peaking, 90
physical education, definition,
2–4
physical fitness, 136
physical well-being, 136
plasma, 28
play, 115–17
players, 118–21
politics and sport, 127–28
posture, 59–62
power, 65, 84–85, 87
prevention of injuries, 97–102
professionalism, 127
protective equipment, 100–101
proteins
for fitness, 92
in diet, 139
pulse, 27

**R**

reaction time, 66, 67, 86
recreation, 116, 117, 133
referees, 121–22
reflexes, 38
rehabilitation, 113
reproductive system, 12
respiratory system, 12, 28, 137
functions of, 28–29, 42
structure and workings, 29–30
reversibility, 68

**S**

shin splints, 112
shoulder injuries, 110
skeletal system, 12, 14
functions of, 14
structure and workings, 14–16
skin system, 12, 40
functions of, 40, 42
injuries, 104
structure and workings, 41
smoke-free generation, 148
smoking
and health, 147–48
society and sport, 114
sociology of sport, 115
soft tissue injuries, 104–8

specificity, 68, 89
spectators, 2, 122–23
and violence, 123–25
speed, 66, 85, 87
spinal cord, 37
Spitz, Mark, 6, 9–10, 129
sponsors, 125–26
sport defined, 115–16
sporting heroes, 2, 6–10, 120
sport in Britain, 114
Sports Council, 114, 115, 130–1,
134–35
sports injuries, 95–97, 104–13
stimulants, 150
stitch, 106
Stoke Mandeville Games, 131
stomach, 32
strength, 65, 74–77, 87
subcutaneous fat, 40

**T**

taping, 101
taste, 32
tendons, 19
injuries, 106, 107
Thompson, Daley, 10
Thorpe, Jim, 7
training for performance, 88–92
methods, 99–100

**U**

umpires, 121–22
urinary system, 34–35

**V**

veins, 25, 27
vena cava, 25
ventricles, 24, 26
vertebra, 15, 16
vitamins
and fitness, 93
in diet, 139–41

**W**

warm-up, 88
water
and fitness, 92
in diet, 141, 144–45
water resistance and motion, 55
weight control, 145–46
Weismuller, Johnny, 8
wetsuits, 101
winding, 111
women and sport, 128
wounds, 102–104